The Interactions between Serotonin and Dopamine in the Compulsive and Impulsive Behavior Underlying Obsessive Compulsive Disorder

Marianne S. Torres-Malaga

Marianne Sierra Torres-Malaga

Copyright © 2018 Marianne Sierra Torres-Malaga

All rights reserved.

ISBN: 1987733304
ISBN-13: 978-1987733303

DEDICATION

THIS WAS PRESENTED AS A PH.D. THESIS AND DEDICATED TO:

MY DAD, WHOSE IMPRESSIVE ACADEMIC ACCOMPLISHMENTS PLANTED THE SEED TO GERMINATE POSTERITY AND SPUR ME TO ACTUALIZE THE LEGACY.

MY HUSBAND, WHO CULTIVATED THE OPPORTUNITY TO FLOURISH AND FOR BEING MY PERSONAL ATM.

MY MOM, FOR WHOM THIS TOPIC INSTRUMENTALLY NOURISHED THE APPEAL TO BE A PART OF THE SOLUTION.

TO **ALL THREE**, OF WHICH IN THEIR OWN WAY HAVE SELFLESSLY HELPED ME TO HARVEST THE ABUNDANCE OF BLESSINGS.

Marianne Sierra Torres-Malaga

CONTENTS

	Dedication	iii
1	Abstract	Pg 7
2	Introduction	Pg 8
3	Literature Review	Pg 40
4	Methodology	Pg 94
5	Compilation of Findings	Pg 101
6	Discussion	Pg 146
7	Hypothesis	Pg 287
8	Conclusion and Recommendations	Pg 293
9	References	Pg 387
	About the Author	Pg 409

1 ABSTRACT

A review of various studies has indicated the efficacy of serotonin (5-hydroxytryptamine [5-HT]) uptake inhibitors such as clomipramine, fluoxetine, fluvoxamine and dopamine in obsessive compulsive disorder (OCD) patients. The role of dopamine (DA) in the pathophysiology of OCD is explored and evidence-based involvement of DA in the pathophysiology of patients who have chronic tic disorder or Tourette's syndrome is presented. Evidence shows that OCD patients with a comorbid chronic tic disorder may have a preferential response to the combination of a DA antagonist with fluvoxamine. Serotonin reuptake inhibitors play a role in the treatment of OCD; preliminary data from the addition of low-dose DA agonists to ongoing 5-HT uptake inhibitors have produced encouraging results.

2 INTRODUCTION

Obsessive compulsive disorder (OCD) is a psychic disorder characterized by the presence of obsessions and compulsions that affects from 1 to 3% of children and adults in the world without distinctions of culture or geography. According to the World Health Organization (WHO), OCD would be included among the main causes of disability in the developing world, ranking in eighth place among the main causes of illness in the adult population of developed countries (Weber et al. 2009). Obsessions are thoughts, images or impulses that the individual recognizes as illogical or unnecessary, and that reach their consciousness involuntarily, causing discomfort and anguish. Despite the lack of control, the individual can recognize that they originate in their own mental processes. Obsessions can be simple repetitive words, thoughts, fears, memories, images or detailed dramatic scenes.

Compulsions are acts that respond to an obligation internally perceived to follow certain rituals or rules, and that also cause functional deterioration. They can be motivated directly by obsessions or by efforts to ward off certain thoughts, impulses, and fears. They lead to elaborate a variety of precise rules for the chronology, speed-rhythm, order, duration and number of repetitions of said acts (American Psychiatric Association, 2000). The individual also sees them as unnecessary, excessive or illogical and involuntary or forced. Children often report compulsions without the perception of a mental component.

The treatment of obsessive compulsive disorder (OCD) can present a challenge for clinical psychiatrists. It is estimated that 1.3% of the population suffers from this disease every year, and 2.7% do so at some point in their lives. The symptoms consist of the appearance of obsessions and compulsions, and although any of these is sufficient to establish the diagnosis, it is common for patients to suffer both. Obsessions are repetitive and stereotyped thoughts that provoke anxiety or anguish and are usually experienced as intrusive or egodystonic phenomena generally recognized as excessive or unrealistic (what distinguishes them from delusions, although in severe cases the difference becomes less clear) (Arntz, Voncken, & Goosen, 2007). Compulsions are ritual actions that are carried out to mitigate the anguish, often in response to obsessions. Obsessions and typical compulsions are, for example, concern for contamination, with rituals and repeated washing, the fear of hurting oneself or others with control rituals or the need for symmetry and order (with the compulsion to order and accommodate objects). OCD can be treated with pharmacotherapy, specialized psychotherapy, treatments directed towards specific anatomical points or the combination of these. The first line of treatment includes cognitive-behavioral therapy (CBT) and pharmacotherapy with selective serotonin reuptake inhibitors (SSRIs). There are three major essential elements when it comes to differentiating the touch of other disorders. The three basic criteria used to make the differential diagnosis of OCD are (Berridge et al. 2005):

1. The essential criterion is functional deterioration as a consequence of the symptoms.
2. Feeling of being forced or invaded by symptoms.
3. The individual recognizes the illogical and excessive nature of these thoughts or acts in some time. (This parameter does not apply to children.)

The validity of the fact that these patients recognize their acts as unnecessary or their thoughts as illogical has been questioned and seems to be somewhat inconsistent since it has been seen in severely deteriorated patients who doubt the need to perform their rituals, while others are convinced of their need to almost psychotic proportions. In fact, the DSM IV has modified the criteria for OCD, so that the awareness of the illogical and excessive symptoms should only be present at some stage of the disease. In children, this criterion does not apply.

Causes of Obsessive Compulsive Disorder

There are probably many causes of Obsessive

Compulsive Disorder. No specific causes have yet been identified, and it may be that OCD is simply a way of responding to the brain with multiple problems. This response is similar to the unique and limited way of the intestines to produce diarrhea when it reacts to a wide variety of problems such as bacterial infections, parasites, contaminated food, anxiety and poor absorption of food (Blier, Habib, & Flament, 2006). However, one thing is clear: OCD is a biological disease of the brain. Let us add to this biological element, the environmental factors that also fulfill their role in OCD. Therefore, even if the true causes of OCD are not well understood, a mixture of both environmental and biological factors seems to be the ones that produce it. Some of the best-known causes are described in the following. The cause that seems to be best understood is that which is related to biochemical factors.

Anatomical factors

Injuries to certain areas of the brain can produce the

symptoms of OCD. Through CT scans, magnetic resonance and positron emission tomography, several abnormalities can be localized in the prefrontal cortex and other areas of the brain (Boulougouris, Chamberlain, & Robbins, 2009). Some studies show an increase or decrease in metabolic activity in various parts of the brain. Other studies show defects in one of the electrical circuits that transmit nerve impulses to various parts of the brain.

Biochemical factors

The brain is obviously a very complex structure. It contains billions of nerve cells (neurons) that communicate and work together. They communicate through electrical signals from one nerve cell to another. Some chemicals, called neurotransmitters, transmit electrical messages from one neuron to another. Neurotransmitters travel from the "end" of a nerve cell (the messenger) to the "start" of another cell (the receptor), through microscopic spaces filled with fluid between cells called synapses. In OCD, there are several neurotransmitters that play an important role: dopamine, serotonin, glutamate and possibly others (Campbell et al. 1999). Evidence shows that serotonin is a key element in OCD. The drugs that affect the serotonin system produce an improvement in the symptoms of OCD. Children who receive serotonin in certain areas of the brain (i.e., caudal core) show improvement in OCD symptoms.

In OCD there seems to be a problem in the serotonin levels or damage in the receiving place blocking or preventing the transmission of electrical messages. A decrease of dopamine in the basal ganglia was also noted when OCD was present. Dopamine also plays an important role in OCD. Hence, psychiatrists prescribe drugs that work on the levels of serotonin and dopamine (Choi, 2009). Oxytocin and glutamate also play an important role. Some adults with OCD report high levels of cerebrospinal fluid and oxytocin. Some patients with Tourette syndrome show low levels of cerebrospinal fluid and oxytocin.

Streptococcal infections

Some children develop symptoms of OCD after suffering a streptococcal bacterial infection. This reaction has been seen in 10-20% of children who develop OCD. It seems that there was an autoimmune disorder since by attacking the bacteria they also attack the basal ganglia of the brain (Davidson, 2003). This condition is called "pediatric autoimmune neuropsychiatric disorder associated with streptococcal infections." A condition similar to liver disease after a streptococcal infection has also been seen.

Neuropsychological factors

Studies show that there are significant problems in the visual-spatial integration of children with OCD. There are also problems with reasoning and memory.

Genetic factors

Although there are clear examples of family members who suffer from OCD, especially parents and their children, studies on the relationship of the genetic link with a special gene have yielded unclear results.

Environmental factors

Very low on the list of causes of OCD is the knowledge of environmental changes of any kind - changes in housing, other medical illnesses, the death of a loved one, pregnancy, problems in school, relationship problems and other stressors of life; all of which can lead to the onset of OCD symptoms.

Prevalence and Epidemiology

The prevalence of OCD in childhood and youth should be understood in the context of the prevalence of subclinical obsessions and compulsions in this group of the population. It was found when interviewing parents of children under 6 years of age, that the urgency to perform acts until "feeling good" and concern with symmetry and rules was very common; these interests decrease when the child moves to school age. Another study in 1997 used self-administered surveys in 1,083 children in grades 4, 6 and 8 (Dell'Osso et al.

2010). Sixty percent of fourth-grade children reported guilty concerns about the lies and a strong tendency to be tested, while fifty percent reported fear of contamination and germs. In eighth grade, concerns in these respects decreased to forty percent, but sixty percent of them reported concerns with cleanliness and fifty percent noticed intrusive aggressive thoughts (Dell'Osso et al. 2010). It was found that these behaviors and symptoms decrease with age.

There are significant disparities and varied methods in the studies, establishing a prevalence of 0.5-3% in adults and since it is already certain that OCD of children and adults is the same disorder, these studies are perfectly applicable to children. The prevalence ranges among children populations in different studies have been 0.2%, 1.2% and more recently a prevalence point of 0.35% was found with an average prevalence of 0.4% (Dell'Osso et al. 2010). Epidemiological studies in adults range from 0.5-3%, but since structured or non-clinical interviews are used exclusively, they can be unreliable and the results may vary according to the clinical criteria considered. Current valid studies estimate the prevalence around 1%.

Valid studies suggest that the sex distribution of OCD continues to be a reflection of clinical samples, where men and women are equally affected, but men are earlier in age. This has been corroborated with some studies where it was found that 35% of men had the onset of symptoms between 5 and 15 years, compared to 20% beginning in this age range among the female group. In addition, men have a longer duration of the disorder before seeking care (Dell'Osso et al. 2010). Generally, the symptoms exist on average 5-8 years before receiving clinical attention. Typically, the patient experiences obsessions and compulsions. Few individuals have one of the two, and if so, cases tend to be obsessions. The type of content is very broad and may vary over time, but reports in adolescents suggest that the most common are related to dirt and germs, fear of a disease suffered by a loved one, accuracy or symmetry and religious scruples. Body functioning, lucky numbers, fear of self-injury, and sexual and aggressive concerns are less common. In adults, the frequency of these categories is similar, except that aggressive and sexual obsessions are more common.

Although a compulsion may originate in any action, only a few are common. A cohort of adolescents showed, in descending order of frequency- cleansing rituals, repetitive actions (do's and don'ts) and verification rituals more commonly. Far fewer subjects report rituals to protect themselves from illnesses or injuries, order maneuvers and counting behaviors. In adults, the most common compulsions are those of verification and cleaning or doing things by numbers, which has been reported as the third most common (Dell'Osso et al. 2010). The analysis of symptoms in independent studies suggests strong reasons to consider a division of OCD into four subgroups: 1. Aggressive, sexual, religious and somatic obsessions with checking compulsions. 2. Symmetry obsessions with compulsions of counting, arranging, ordering and repeating. 3. Obsessions of contamination with compulsions of washing and cleaning. 4.

Obsessions of hoarding with compulsions of hoarding and collecting. The researchers propose that the course, genetic risk, neuropathology, and treatment may be different between these subgroups and that this subdivision admits new analyzes. For example, it has been suggested that the genetic locus model has greater support in families with symptoms of order and symmetry, but the response to SSRIs does not support the difference in response between the groups. It should be considered that in this classification, other symptoms have been excluded and that these change in the course of the disease.

In other areas of functioning, children with OCD are more selectively impaired than the general population. Academic performance and extracurricular functioning are often preserved, although the quality of relationships with peers may vary. Studies in adults indicate important impairment in the role and social function, and the severity of the disorder is correlated with the degree of social deterioration (den Heuvel et al. 2010). Consistent studies of children in treatment programs have shown average intellectual quotients, but the selection biases of these cohorts should be taken into account for this analysis. Severe symptoms can involve patients and their families completely. It is common to learn wash rituals that consume up to four hours a day; spending a whole bar of soap on each session; leaving hands looking rough, macerated and dramatically increasing monthly water bills. The compulsions of counting and ordering can spend up to half a day producing quite a severe disturbance. Repetitive rituals performed at night can last until dawn, shortening the sleep time by several hours. Verification and cleaning rituals can cause physical damage, such as skin lacerations, ulcerations, and chemical burns.

The reaction of the family to the patient's symptoms is crucial. Many common responses from parents can cause delays in the evaluation and treatment of childhood OCD. Although patients are embarrassed and hide the content and limitations imposed by their symptoms, severe deterioration rarely escapes family members. Parents may delay obtaining treatment because of a false hope that the symptoms will disappear if everyone agrees and collaborates in the execution of activities. This type of assistance from the family does not alleviate the child's anxiety (Denys et al. 2004). Many parents have difficulty getting rid of themselves in these rituals. Children can exhort, implore, or use other means to compel their parents to collaborate; children and parents can become pathologically entangled in rituals. Parents may not understand that their children suffer from a serious disorder despite their normal development in other areas. In addition, there is the manifestation of children that thoughts or acts are ridiculous or unnecessary; this can give a false security to parents who think that this is only a stage. This may be reinforced by parents with subclinical obsessions or behaviors similar to compulsive ones, who may not recognize symptoms in their child. The neglect of clinicians and pediatricians who are not well acquainted with the disorder can lead to erroneous symptoms such as normal reactions. It is a feared and painful moment when parents recognize that their child has lost control of their thoughts and actions.

Four discoveries have revived research on OCD since the decade of the 1980's. First, that serotonin reuptake inhibitor medication is effective for the treatment of many of the patients with OCD. Subsequently, powerful techniques were applied for the observation of brain structures and measurement of regional brain activity, in order to understand how this happened (Dougherty Rauch & Jenike, 2004). At the same time, some studies have focused on the prevalence of OCD. Finally, attention has been focused on the genetic transmission of OCD. These investigations have allowed researchers to deepen their understanding of the prevalence, etiology, course, and pathology of these symptoms and extend the knowledge of basic brain structures and functions.

The observation that serotonin (5-HT) reuptake inhibitors improve obsessive compulsive disorder (OCD) was the first indication that 5-HT could play an important role in this anxiety disorder. The first drug of this type to be used was chlorimipramine or clomipramine, the efficacy of which has been demonstrated in open and double-blinded studies (Hollander 2005). Clomipramine has a high affinity for the 5-HT reuptake site and low affinity for the corresponding noradrenaline site (NA). However, its metabolite - desmethylchlorimipramine - predominantly inhibits NA reuptake. Therefore, clomipramine cannot be regarded as a true selective serotonin reuptake inhibitor (SSRI) when administered chronically.

However, other evidence has strengthened the hypothesis of serotonergic mediation of anti-OCD drug action. The first was the finding that imipramine is much less effective than clomipramine in OCD. This difference contrasts with the equivalence of the therapeutic action of the two drugs in unipolar depressive disorder and the moderate advantage of clomipramine over imipramine in panic disorder. Because imipramine also inhibits 5-HT and NA reuptake, its ineffectiveness in OCD indicates that inhibition of NA reuptake is unnecessary or even counterproductive. The second evidence became known with the introduction of SSRIs, such as fluoxetine, fluvoxamine, and sertraline, whose metabolites do not interfere with NA reuptake. Such compounds were also found to be effective in the treatment of OCD.

Pathophysiology of OCD

Judith Rapoport who adopted the perspective of evolutionary psychology formulated the most accepted theory of OCD pathophysiology (Joel & Avisar, 2001). Based on Charles Darwin, this theoretical orientation postulates that the behavioral characteristics of animals are subject to natural selection in the same way as anatomical and physiological ones. Realizing that the most frequent compulsions are cleaning and checking if doors and windows are closed, Rapoport has hypothesized that such manifestations would be exaggerations of self-cleaning routines (self-grooming) and to confer territorial demarcations, respectively (Joel, Doljansky, & Schiller, 2005). These were acquired by numerous species because of the adaptive value to prevent disease and to guarantee living space needed for feeding and reproduction. In the author's expression, the compulsion to repeatedly wash hands was nothing more than a *"grooming gone wild,"* that is, an exacerbation of self-cleaning behavior.

This conception about the genesis of OCD led to the search for behaviors with compulsive characteristics in animals, two of which attracted attention. The first is the habit of dogs, especially those of the Labrador breed, to lick excessively the paws, which causes serious injuries. This condition is called "acral dermatitis." The second is the behavior, which occurs in certain birds subjected to captivity, of incessantly removing the feathers with the beak. If such behaviors are homology with a compulsive disorder, i.e. sharing the same neurobiological substrate, they should be equally susceptible to SSRIs. This prediction was confirmed in controlled pharmacological trials, resulting in treatment of choice for these conditions. This is probably the only example of a veterinary treatment that derived from a theory about the pathophysiology of a psychiatric disorder of the human being.

Biological Basis

Deregulation of neurotransmitters: One theory about the biological basis of panic disorder is that there is an initial excess of noradrenaline, causing down-regulation of post-synaptic adrenergic receptors. This theory is supported by evidence that patients with panic disorder are hypersensitive to alpha 2 antagonists and hyposensitive to alpha 2 agonists. Thus, yohimbine, alpha 2 antagonist, acts as a promoter of NA release by cutting off the "brake cable" of the presynaptic NA auto-receptor. The consequence of administration of yohimbine is the occurrence of an exaggerated response in patients with panic disorder, including the precipitation of typical attacks. Caffeine is also panicogenic. That is, caffeine is an antagonist of adenosine that amplifies the action of second-messengers of noradrenaline; when patients receive a caffeine dose equivalent to four or six cups of coffee, many experience a panic attack, which is not the case with most normal people. On the other hand, patients with panic disorder present a decreased physiological response to post-synaptic adrenergic agonists, perhaps as a consequence of the hyperactive noradrenergic system.

The neurotransmitter GABA (gamma-aminobutyric acid) and its allosteric modulation by benzodiazepines have been implicated in the biological basis of panic disorder. That is, it appears that the ability of benzodiazepines to modulate GABA would be out of balance. This could be due to changes in the amounts of endogenous benzodiazepines (ie "the brain's own alprazolam" or "a diazepam-like compound") or changes in the sensitivity of the benzodiazepine receptor itself. Very little is known about endogenous benzodiazepine binders so more emphasis has been placed on the investigation of benzodiazepine receptor responsiveness in patients with panic disorder. However, it is possible that the brain synthesizes less than the amount required of the total endogenous agonist; thus, there would be less ability of the brain to reduce anxiety by its own means due to the supposed deficiency of the naturally occurring total benzodiazepine agonist. On the other hand, it is possible that the brain is producing excess anxiogenic inverse agonists, leading the patient with panic disorder to experience more anxiety and panic attacks due to this alleged undesired increase in naturally occurring benzodiazepine inverse agonist.

These are only theoretical possibilities, but some data indeed suggest benzodiazepine receptor abnormality in patients with panic disorder, in which the "point of sensitivity" is shifted towards the confirmation of the inverse agonist. Conceptually, the resting state of the benzodiazepine receptor complex - GABA A - chloride channel is shifted to the left in the spectrum of the agonists already discussed. Thus, the conductance of the chloride channel is already too low for the altered sensitivity of the benzodiazepine receptor site. Evidence for this arises from the fact that such patients require the administration of exogenous benzodiazepine binders (i.e., alprazolam or clonazepam) to bring the point the sensitivity of the receptor complex back to normal. In addition, flumazenil, which is neutral, and without behavioral effects in normal individuals because it acts as a relatively pure antagonist, acts differently in patients with panic disorder. In these patients, flumazenil acts as an inverse agonist because of the abnormal deviation of the point of sensitivity towards the confirmation of the inverse agonist. Thus, although flumazenil acts as an antagonist without behavioral effects in the normal individual, it acts as a partial inverse agonist in patients with panic disorder and causes panic attacks in these patients.

Hypersensitivity to carbon dioxide: Another theory involving the biological substrate of panic disorder is based on the observations that patients with this disorder experience attacks more readily (than people without the disorder) when they inhale carbon dioxide or when they receive lactate. This gave rise to the theory of hypersensitivity to carbon dioxide in patients with panic disorder, with the consequent hypothesis that these patients demonstrate such findings because they are chronic hyperventilators.

False suffocation alarm theory: This theory proposes that patients with panic disorder have a suffocation monitor located in the brainstem that interprets the signals mistakenly, performing false shots, which would trigger the "false suffocation alarm" (panic attack). Many factors are consistent with this hypothesis, including the earlier theory about chronic hyperventilation and hypersensitivity to carbon dioxide. The Ondina Curse Disorder (central congenital hypoventilation syndrome) appears to be virtually the opposite of panic disorder and is characterized by decreased sensitivity of the choking alarm, causing patients suffering from this disorder do *not* present adequate breathing, especially when asleep. These various observations support the existence of a distinct suffocation monitor, which is hypersensitive to panic disorder and hyposensitive in the Ondina Curse. According to this theory, spontaneous (that is, unexpected) panic attacks would be mediated by this mechanism, although chronic fear or anxiety is not.

Genetic Transmission of OCD

Current evidence suggests genetic transmission of a

vulnerability to OCD in many cases. This is derived from the increase in concordance rats between monozygotic twins compared to the dizygotic ones, and the increase in frequency among first-degree relatives of diagnosed patients. Some researchers have discovered increased frequency of subclinical obsessive compulsive symptoms among first-degree relatives but without a significant increase in OCD levels. Subsequently, another study of a family was conducted using a control group; of 145 first-degree relatives, only one (0.6%) met the diagnostic criteria for OCD. In 1992, a detailed study was carried out with a group of 166 relatives of OCD patients and 182 relatives of subjects of a control group; the rates of OCD in first-degree relatives of both groups were comparable (2.5% vs. 2.3%). However, rats of anxiety disorders were about twice as many in relatives of the first group compared to the control group.

Reports of high OCD rates among patients with La Tourette Syndrome, tics and/or family history of tics in patients with proven OCD, suggest that OCD may be caused by the same genetic etiology as this syndrome; reevaluation of a cohort of the National Mental Health Institute and its relatives in a follow-up of 2-7 years, support this hypothesis. Fifty-seven percent of 54 patients with proven OCD had a history of tics, 15% met criteria for Tourette and 22% had multiple chronic tics. Among their relatives, 14% had a history of diagnosed tics. These findings suggest that future investigations of the course of the disease or the efficacy of treatment should analyze the data according to whether those subjects have had tics and a family history of tics.

EEG studies of children and adults with OCD have shown significant differences with control subjects. Reports of OCD subjects show the decreased latency of rapid eye movements (REM) but normal REM density. This pattern is different from that seen in patients with depression in whom there is a decrease in both the latency and the density of REM. Evoked potentials were made in adults with OCD, finding increases in cortical processing speed that suggest an increase in response in the left hemisphere.

Neuropsychological Processes

The investigations give support to talk about frontal lobe dysfunction in OCD, which affects visuospatial integration, reasoning, and memory, but these data have been found in adults and are not necessarily extrapolated to children. There has been talk that the deficiencies are in the dominant frontal lobe and that the failure in their inhibitory responses explains the dysfunction in the dominant temporal and parietal lobes, but these findings have not been confirmed. Immaturity of frontal lobe functions has been reported in 16 adolescents with OCD, but in another study, 21 children with OCD were examined, without previous medication, and they used a neuropsychological battery without finding abnormalities. CT of adolescents with OCD or OCD subjects with onset of symptoms in adolescence suggests a ventricular enlargement, regardless of age, sex, duration, and types of symptoms. In addition, a decrease in volume was observed mainly in the caudate nucleus bilaterally.

By means of magnetic resonance, adult patients with OCD and normal subjects have been compared, finding abnormalities in frontal cortex, cingulum and lenticular nucleus. The history of medical treatment or family history had no significant influence on the findings. It has been reported that there is an increase in the size of the caudate nucleus, affirming later that the size of the left nucleus exceeded that of the right one. Other authors have not found the significant structural difference between OCD subjects and normal subjects. In 1996, a study was conducted on 10 women with OCD, finding an increase at the opercula level and throughout the cortex, as well as a decrease in all white matter; in a parallel study, they found no difference in a group of 24 adults with OCD, compared with the control group. Changes in regional cerebral blood flow have been observed with xenon inhalation. Subjects who were stressed specifically to increase anxiety showed decreased temporal flow. So far, no PET studies have been published in children with OCD, but two studies of adults report an increase in frontal medial flow.

With technetium taken, increased activity in the orbitofrontal cortex was observed with significant bilateral decrease in activity in the caudate head, a phenomenon previously noted by others.

In the last five years, **Positron** Emission Tomography, also called PET imaging or a PET **scan,** have become the most powerful tool to reach the understanding of OCD. The first wave of studies examined the regional consumption of glucose in the brain of people with OCD compared to controls. These studies report increased activity in the orbital rotation and the caudate nucleus. In another study, individuals with OCD were examined while provoking them with feared stimuli, observing activation in the right caudate, orbital, thalamic and anterior singular rotation. The initial comparison of OCD and depressed adults suggests a bilateral increase in metabolism in the orbital rotation and head of the caudate nucleus, thus it was proposed that the orbital rotation could be specific for tension and anxiety in OCD, but the increase in activity was not confirmed of the caudate nucleus. It has also been observed that adult patients with OCD of documented beginning in adolescence had increased bilateral prefrontal activity and in the anterior single turn, which was interpreted as a fronto-limbic-basal circuit. Increased metabolism in premotor and medial frontal regions was reported in obsessive slowness.

Subsequent studies studied brain metabolic changes after treatment with medication and behavioral therapy. In the case of clomipramine, eight patients were examined after treatment and it was found that the activity of the left caudate and orbital frontal cortex decreased. Regarding fluoxetine, concomitant with cognitive behavioral therapy, it was found that in the responders there was a decrease in the metabolism of glucose in the right caudate. It was also found that adults with OCD beginning in childhood, showed decreased orbitofrontal metabolism related to both medication and the spontaneous improvement of OCD with severe ranges. Ten subjects were studied during the provocation of symptoms and elevated activity was found in the medial orbitofrontal cortex, lateral, frontal and anterior single rotation, as well as in the insular cortex, caudate lenticular (putamen and global palidus) and amygdala.

Spectroscopic Functional Magnetic Resonance

Spectroscopic Functional Magnetic Resonance is a non-invasive technique that studies brain function using magnetic fields, which are applied to determine the density and activity of glutamate and N-acetyl-aspartate (a marker of injury and neuronal damage) in the brain. In 2000, eleven children with OCD without medication were studied and a decrease was described in these levels in the caudate nuclei bilaterally. In addition, Rosenberg (2000) found that after treatment with paroxetine, these levels in the caudate were normal. Taken together, structural studies suggest differences between patients with OCD and healthy in the frontal cortex and caudate nucleus. These findings are corroborated by more detailed functional studies that show high activity in the orbitofrontal, frontal lateral and single turn regions and in the caudate and lenticular nuclei (putamen and globus pallidus).

More recent work has focused on glutamate receptors in the caudate and decreased neuronal activity in medial thalamus. Taking other neuroanatomical studies and these findings, a great consensus has emerged that functional defects in a cortico-striato-thalamocortical circuit define OCD.

3 LITERATURE REVIEW

Serotonin

Serotonin is an organic compound found primarily in blood. In 1948, serotonin was partially purified, crystallized and named. In 1948, a substance with a vasoconstrictor nature was isolated for the first time in serum, which was called serotonin ($C_{10}H_{12}N_2O$). This agent was subsequently chemically identified as 5-hydroxytryptamine (5-HT) and has since been associated with a wide range of physiological properties. It later discovered that serotonin is widely found in all nature, as well as in other parts of the body besides blood. Serotonin was also found in wasp stings, scorpion venom and a variety of foods such as pineapple, banana, plums, walnuts, turkey, ham, milk and cheese. In addition, serotonin has been found in the human gut, platelets, and brain. Serotonin plays a role in the body, as it is a neurotransmitter in the brain. The lack of serotonin in the body can result in lack of rational emotion, feelings of irritability and loss, crying crises, sleep disorders and a host of other emotional problems. For our purpose, we understand that Serotonin is a substance called a neurotransmitter and exists naturally in our brain. Its function is to drive the transmission from one nerve cell (neuron) to another. Chemically, serotonin, or 5-hydroxytryptamine (5-HT), is an indolamine product of the transformation of the amino acid L-Tryptophan.

5-HT is a neurotransmitter monoamine synthesized mainly in two areas: centrally, in the serotonergic neurons of the nuclei located in the brainstem, and peripherally, in the intestinal enterochromaffin cells and in the serotonergic neurons of the mesenteric plexus. In plasma, serotonin travels stored within platelets (Sirek and Sirek, 1970). The functions of serotonin are very diverse. For example, it plays an important role in regulating appetite through satiety, balancing sexual health, controlling body temperature, motor activity and perceptual and cognitive functions (Heninger, 1997). In addition, it intervenes with other neurotransmitters in the development of depression, anxiety, anxiety, fear or aggression (Pihl and LeMarquand, 1998, Albert and Benkelfat, 2013).

Serotonin is also necessary to make melatonin, which regulates sleep and has an important role in bone density and architecture. It also intervenes in the inhibition of gastric secretion, the stimulation of the smooth muscle and the secretion of hormones by the pituitary gland. It even plays an important role in the lymphocyte proliferation depending on the type of stimulated receptor (Cooper et al., 1996; Fink et al., 1999).

Serotonin is a neurotransmitter produced by the human body. Neurotransmitters are substances that help transmit chemical signals from one neuron to the next. There are several types of neurotransmitters with different functions in our body. Serotonin is a chemical substance responsible for maintaining the balance of our mood. The levels we present of this neurotransmitter have a direct relationship with our well-being and happiness. One of the main functions of serotonin is to contribute to the proper functioning of a person's body. It is responsible for establishing the levels of sexual desire in men and women and also has a responsibility for our reactions to

Effects of Serotonin and Dopamine in Obsessive Compulsive Disorder

situations that generate stress. When a situation presents an individual with pressure, their response to this event can show what serotonin does. It sends the neurons the necessary information so that you can resolve that sensation that gives you some discomfort, in the same way, serotonin produces in the human body melatonin, which is a substance that is responsible for regulating normal sleep cycles.

Serotonin is synthesized from the essential amino acid tryptophan in a short metabolic pathway that involves two enzymes: tryptophan hydroxylase (TPH), which catalyzes the limiting step, and an aromatic L-amino acid decarboxylase (DDC). There are two isoforms of TPH- TPH1, located in several tissues, and TPH2, which is brain-specific (Walther and Bader, 2003). Once synthesized, serotonin passes into the blood, where it is captured by platelets. Intracellular calcium plays a regulatory role in this process (Camilleri and Von der Ohe, 1994). In serotonergic neurons, 5-HT is secreted from the terminal buttons and along the entire axon to the synaptic space. The neurons of the raphe nuclei are the main source of

5-HT release in the brain. These nuclei innervate almost all areas of the central nervous system, including the hypothalamus, where serotonin acts as a signal of satiety (Leibowitz, 1986, Sugrue, 1987, Curzon, 1990) and regions related to anxiety, depression, and impulsivity (Haleem, 2006; Fineberg et al., 2010). From the synaptic space, 5-HT is free to diffuse, activate serotonergic receptors and regain.

Amino Acids that Promote the Natural Production of Serotonin

Three of the most commonly used serotonin supplements are the amino acids tryptophan, 5-HTP, and SAM-e.

Tryptophan

Tryptophan is an amino acid par excellence. It reaches your body thanks to the consumption of proteins of animal origin, and this helps in the process of synthesizing serotonin in the digestive system, providing many benefits at the time of digestion of meals. It is important that you regulate the amounts of these foods that give you tryptophan; you must maintain a balance and not allow excesses.

5-HTP (5-hydroxytryptophan)

5-HTP comes from a plant native to Africa; to obtain its benefits, its seeds are used. It is an ally of tryptophan. The important thing to consider about supplements is that it is indicated by a certified doctor, is necessary to be oriented to your needs, and familiarizing yourself with these terms that can be a bit difficult. Those are key to keeping you up-to-date with your health needs.

SAM-e (s-adenosylmethionine)

SAM-e is an excellent motivator of metabolism; that is, it also helps a person lose weight. This supplement is produced naturally by each of the body's cells; thus, many researchers around the world have implemented it to treat depression, achieving excellent results. It is a mixture that is related to the release of serotonin in our body.

Vitamins and Minerals That Increase Serotonin

Serotonin in Vitamins

Serotonin plays a key role in the central nervous system, which is why the B vitamins are classified as essential in the production of serotonin. These vitamins are:

1. Vitamin B6 (Pyridoxine): It is a water-soluble vitamin, which means that when it fulfills its function in the body, is discarded naturally through the urine. It must be present to facilitate the conversion of 5-HTP or tryptophan to serotonin.
2. Vitamin B9 (folic acid): In our body, its presence is necessary for the formation of structural proteins and to maintain optimal levels of hemoglobin. It is proven that when the level of folic acid in the blood is low, serotonin levels are also low.
3. Vitamin C: The presence of vitamin C in our body is of vital importance in metabolic reactions. In addition to this, consuming the daily dose could increase serotonin

levels. Similarly, there are investigations that place it as a natural antidepressant.

4. <u>Vitamin D</u>: It plays a very important role in the formation of our bones and teeth. It favors the absorption of calcium at the time of digestion, and in the same way, it is related to cell rejuvenation. It is related to serotonin because the deficiency of both causes depression in people.

5. <u>Magnesium</u>: This is presented as an essential component in all detoxification processes of our body. It also helps to balance the levels of serotonin, as it has been revealed in many studies reveal that it has great potentialities in the recovery of patients with psychiatric disorders.

6. <u>Zinc</u>: It is a mineral considered essential in our body. It lodges in our muscles, hair, and bones, generating considerable improvements. When it fulfills its proper function, it is disposed of from the body in a natural way and it helps in the correct absorption of serotonin.

Herbs that Increase Serotonin Levels

Nowadays, everything related to the increase of serotonin in a natural way through herbs or plants is in the public domain. Surely, access to these will depend on where a person is and their resources. The way an individual wants to consume it will also depend on the indications of your specialist physician and your creativity.

Curcumin (Curcuma longa)

Curcumin is a herbaceous silver native to India and has many healing properties. It also has the advantage of producing dopamine and serotonin, and studies have revealed that the human body absorbs it better when it is previously mixed with black pepper.

Garcinia cambogia

Garcinia cambogia is an acidic fruit that has its origins in the Asian continent and is made up of almost 200 varieties worldwide. It has many therapeutic uses, one of which is that when the juice of this fruit is mixed with L-Carnitine, it is a powerful burner of fats that promote weight loss; also, it increases serotonin levels.

Rhodiola Rosea

Rhodiola Rosea is a small plant with flowers that develop in any cold area of the world. It is proven by researchers that this natural medicine has a large number of adaptogens and its infusion helps to control depression in women who have suffered severe cases of postpartum depression. It is an excellent option to raise serotonin levels and combat stress.

Foods That Increase It Naturally

There is a wide variety of foods that are aimed at people who have low levels of this chemical. These foods must contain tryptophan, which is the amino acid par excellence that helps serotonin to perform the functions that correspond. Proteins of animal origin are the most indicated to obtain this amino acid. You must consume fresh fish, beef, chicken or lamb, eggs, milk, and bananas, and maintain an adequate balance in the portions.

Climbing serotonin levels with physical exercise

Throughout the day, a person should always think about giving their body a moment. Exercising just 45 minutes a day, doing any physical activity that you choose, helps increase the levels of serotonin, which gives a feeling of self-satisfaction. For example, daily walking with constancy brings great benefits to the cardiovascular system. It is estimated that walking half an hour, three times a week and at a sustained speed, improves the performance of the heart. Doing a little physical activity not only stimulates the production of serotonin, but also benefits the metabolism, increases its capacity to produce energy, and therefore, it better consumes the adipose deposits (or fat) lodged in the body, and subsequently allows you to lose weight.

The connection between Serotonin and Mental Illness

Serotonin has also been called "the happiness hormone" because of its qualities related to providing well-being, improving self-esteem, relaxing and helping to concentrate. Many of the alterations in their levels affect our mental health in different ways. Thus, given the functions performed in our body, the drugs that interact with it are used in multiple disorders. Some of these disorders are depression, phobia or social anxiety, obsessive compulsive disorder, panic disorder, intermittent explosive disorder, dementia, and serotonin syndrome. It is common for these disorders to have specific cognitive deficits, so in some cases, it is advisable to perform a neuropsychological assessment to help recognize the strengths and weaknesses. Usually, the first step of any diagnosis or intervention is to evaluate if there is a problem in the main cognitive functions.

Depression and its relationship with Serotonin Levels

It is believed that depression is caused by an imbalance in serotonin levels. The process involved is the neuronal regeneration, in which it is involved. According to the neurologist Barry Jacobs, depression occurs when there is not enough neuronal regeneration. SSRI antidepressants (selective serotonin reuptake inhibitors) help produce new brain cells and boost mood. Although it would be ideal to be able to measure their levels in the brain, this is not possible. Despite this, we can measure certain blood levels and it has been shown to be lower in individuals with depression. Unfortunately, if a low level is found, it is unclear if it was from baseline, from before the depression, or as a result of the decrease in serotonin. In fact, it is known that SSRI and SSRI antidepressants (selective serotonin and noradrenaline reuptake inhibitors) work, but not the *why*.

Social Anxiety and its relationship with Serotonin

Imbalances in the levels of this neurotransmitter could cause the appearance of disorders related to anxiety. Some of these are panic disorder, obsessive compulsive disorder, social anxiety or social phobia, generalized anxiety disorder, and more. It is not clear if what produces the anxious symptoms is a deficit or an excess of this neurotransmitter. Until now, it was believed that low levels of serotonin were the cause, but recent research seems to deny it. JAMA Psychiatry has published that people suffering from social anxiety have higher than normal levels. Moreover, the University of Uppsala has shown that in the amygdala (brain structure involved in fear), there is an excess of serotonin in patients with social anxiety. Of course, this can be exclusive of the social anxiety disorder, but it will be necessary to continue investigating through research.

Obsessive Compulsive Disorder and its relationship with Serotonin

The relationship of obsessive compulsive disorder (OCD) and this neurotransmitter is given by the influence of SSRI antidepressants in the improvement of the disorder. SSRIs are inhibitors of serotonin reuptake; that is, they are drugs that facilitate their availability so that there are no low levels of the neurotransmitter. Just as a cold is not caused by a deficit in acetylsalicylic acid, we cannot say that OCD is produced by a deficit of this substance. However, it seems that it fulfills some function in the course of the disorder. Deficits of this serotonin aggregate with symptoms such as low mood, impulsiveness, and aggressiveness.

Panic Disorder and Serotonin Levels

The cause of panic disorder, as was already the case in OCD, is unknown. Although low levels of serotonin have been found in patients suffering from panic attacks, it is not known which came first. The only thing we know is that SSRIs also work in the case of people suffering from panic disorder. For the time being, and until there is more research in this regard, we know that those psychotropic drugs that contain it, help to improve anxious symptoms in general, and those of panic attacks in particular.

Intermittent Explosive Disorder and Serotonin

The intermittent explosive disorder is a behavior disorder characterized by explosions of unwarranted anger. Serotonin is a neurotransmitter that helps regulate mood and help reduce these attacks in number and intensity. For this reason, the pharmacological treatments for this disorder are SSRI antidepressants that interact with this neurotransmitter. The intermittent explosive disorder is considered to be incurable. However, one can treat the patient through psychotherapy and medication, so that the aggressive behavior, and the feeling of frustration and internal anger, is reduced.

Dementia and Low Levels of Serotonin

As a consequence of age, there is a cognitive deterioration associated with the loss of neuronal connections. The activity of neurotransmitters, responsible for the transmission of neuronal information, is reduced. Aging is not synonymous with dementia, although there are cases in which significant cognitive deterioration is observed. The most well-known of dementia is Alzheimer's disease. In an international study published in 2006, researchers from all over the world found a serotonergic deficiency in Alzheimer's patients. They hypothesized that Alzheimer's memory problems are due to a malfunction of serotonin receptors. The receptors are the cells capable of receiving the transmissions of neurotransmitters. There is no evidence to show that increasing serotonin levels prevents or delays Alzheimer's.

Serotonin Deficiency and Depression

There is research related to serotonin being responsible for the different ways in which depression is evidenced; when a person has a low production of this chemical, the main function of being a neurotransmitter, will decrease. What it brings as a consequence is that the person does not have the capacity, or the positive impulse, in any situation of the different areas of daily life. Anxiety, personality disorders, and anger can be related to serotonin and its effects on humans. Although it has never been possible to verify the levels of serotonin in the human brain, it is very true that it is responsible for sending those messages towards the nervous system, and each person will manifest a different behavior and stimulus. It is important to highlight that many times the depression produces physical, painful symptoms, cardiac, and digestive abnormalities, which are said to be physical because the depressed person somatizes the depression.

Serotonin and Postpartum Depression

The natural process of giving life to another human being is often a time that some women would not want to live again; this is due to postpartum depression that is related to the low levels of serotonin in the blood of these women. It is important to know that postpartum depression develops quickly, usually lasts 1 to 3 days after delivery, but can last for months; most women suffer this process, but some cannot overcome it without specialized help. During pregnancy there is a great secretion of endorphins and a hormonal state that favors good mood; serotonin is present in excellent levels, which allows the anxious mother to feel happy. When the birth comes, a hormonal change again originates abruptly, changes the whole family routine, and that encounter with the new reality favors the appearance of postpartum depression. Regarding the treatment or medication, it is recommended to establish the normal values regarding serotonin; that way, a certified specialist can decide if it is necessary to use antidepressants. Anti-depressants are very effective, but they can produce many side effects, especially at the beginning of treatment when your body has not yet become accustomed.

The relationship between Serotonin and Anxiety

Anxiety is an inherent process of the human species, which is why anxiety can be classified as a pathological state with a series of symptoms such as irritability, intolerance to loud noises, mild memory loss, muscle tension and cognitive deficit. Now, serotonin is related to states of anxiety because when there are low levels of this substance, the neurons do not receive an adequate message, and it is at that moment where they begin to observe the symptoms such as anxiety. Anxiety is characterized by manifested alterations in the vegetative nervous system, especially by an increase in the tone of the nervous system, which is responsible for accelerating all the organic processes of our body. This acceleration is often not manifested physically but by the rapidity of mental processes, which cause difficulties to concentrate on conversations or on a specific topic. When the anxiety increases, there are nervous breakdowns.

Serotonin syndrome

An excess of serotonin can be harmful. SSRI antidepressants are considered safe. However, they can cause "Serotonin Syndrome" due to high concentrations of this neurotransmitter. It usually occurs when two drugs (in which serotonin is involved) are used simultaneously. The problems occur when starting with medication or increasing the dose; when using monoamine oxidase ("MAOI's") enzyme inhibitors (an enzyme that degrades serotonin) with SSRIs; or consume LSD or ecstasy. The symptoms are agitation, hallucinations, increased body temperature, tachycardia, sweating, loss of coordination, spasms, nausea, vomiting, diarrhea, and changes in blood pressure. It is not considered dangerous, but it is necessary to treat it in case it results in a serious medical condition. The treatment consists in the withdrawal of the drug, intravenous muscle relaxants, and blockers of serotonin production.

Serotonin Reuptake Inhibitors

SSRIs represent the main strategy for the pharmacological treatment of OCD, due to its proven efficacy and its adequate profile of possible adverse effects. Clomipramine, a tricyclic antidepressant, is effective but is associated with common adverse effects that limit its use. Fluvoxamine was the first SSRI whose efficacy was proven, but there is no evidence that any drug in this group is superior to the others, so the selection should be based on the profile of adverse effects and drug interactions, in addition to the preference from the patients. The greater efficacy of SSRIs in OCD is observed at high doses, such as 80 mg of fluoxetine, 40 mg of escitalopram, 300 mg of fluvoxamine or 100 mg of paroxetine. The symptoms of OCD usually take longer than those of major depression to respond to monotherapy with SSRIs (at least 8 to 12 weeks). Some individuals report subjective improvement in symptoms more quickly than others, even from the first weeks of treatment.

The US Food and Drug Administration (FDA) has not approved the SSRI citalopram for use in OCD, but the clinicians consider that it is as effective as the others in treating this disease, and historically, it is used for this purpose because of its good tolerability. The FDA warns that at doses above 40 mg daily, this drug could be associated with abnormalities in the electrocardiogram (ECG) and risk of arrhythmia. In elderly people, it is not recommended to administer doses higher than 20 mg daily, and it has been suggested to avoid its use in individuals with a corrected QT interval> 500 ms, or factors that predispose to the appearance of arrhythmias. This effect seems to be less for escitalopram, on which the FDA has not published the same warning. It is suggested to follow up with a routine ECG in all patients who have benefited clinically with the use of citalopram and do not want to change drugs.

The drugs called selective serotonin reuptake inhibitors (SSRIs) are 6: fluoxetine (Prozac, Fluoxeren, Fluoxetine), fluvoxamine (Maveral, Fevarin, Dumirox), paroxetine (Sereupin, Seroxat, Eutimil, Daparox), sertraline (Zoloft, Tatig), citalopram (Elopram, Seropram) and escitalopram (Entact, Cipralex), and are united by a part of their mechanism of action. While SSRIs are effective in treating children and adolescents with OCD, there is no evidence that the administration of high doses is as useful as in adults; also, there is some concern about adverse effects associated with this strategy. The three SSRIs approved to treat children with OCD are fluoxetine (in children> 7 years), sertraline (in> 6 years) and fluvoxamine (in> 8 years); clomipramine has also been approved for this indication in children> 10 years. Clomipramine is a tricyclic antidepressant approved by the FDA for the treatment of OCD; it is the most potent inhibitor of serotonin reuptake of the tricyclic group and, in addition, binds with high affinity to other receptors and reuptake sites. There are indications, based on meta-analysis, in which it could be more effective in treating OCD than SSRIs, but several methodological factors complicate the interpretation of the studies, and those that made direct comparisons did not show superiority.

Within this pharmacological class, the drugs differ not only by their affinity for the serotonin transporter (5HT) but also by their affinity for various other receptors present in the brain cells (see below). These differences are not a trivial matter, but instead, have important implications in terms of both therapeutic effects and unwanted effects. For example, within the same pharmacological class, we find fluoxetine (whose specific affinity for 5HT-2C serotonin receptors is probably at the base of its ability to induce weight loss) and we also find paroxetine (whose affinity for H1 receptors of histamine is the basis of its ability to induce weight gain). Within the same pharmacological class, we find both medicines that can prompt weight gain and medicines able to reduce it. The explanation of these phenomena is found in the details of the mechanism of action.

All SSRIs, when they reach the cells of the central nervous system (neurons), have a variable ability to inhibit, at the level of the presynaptic receptors placed on the neuron, the reabsorption of serotonin. In this way, a greater quantity of serotonin is available in the space between the neurons responsible for the exchange of signals (synapses). This increase triggers a cascade of changes in the target neuron which results in a change in the number and affinity of the serotonergic receptors at this level and, subsequently, in a change in the neuron discharge rate. At this point, the alteration of serotonin levels begins to translate into changes at the symptomatological and behavioral level; the undesirable effects begin to decrease, and the anxiolytic and antidepressant effects appear according to the main characteristics of each molecule.

The ability of each individual SSRI to inhibit the reuptake of serotonin is variable as the affinity of the single drug to the other receptors on the cells of the central nervous system varies. In substance, from one medicine to another, both the ability to modify the levels of serotonin and the ability to modify the levels of other neuro mediators present in the central nervous system change with different effects on behavior. In a series of recent works, radioactive ligands were used to trace the receptor profile and affinity of each individual SSRI for the different receptors and carriers present in the brain. As an example of such work, escitalopram and fluoxetine have been shown to be potent and selective inhibitors of the serotonin transporter, with escitalopram being the most selective. Paroxetine and sertraline have been shown to be poorly selective inhibitors having a fair affinity, as well as for 5HT, dopamine and norepinephrine transporters. Sertraline has shown an ability to inhibit 5HT transporters, comparable to escitalopram and fluoxetine while being less selective than the latter. Fluoxetine has a moderate but absolutely specific affinity for 5HT-2C serotonin receptors. Fluvoxamine was poorly selective, demonstrating an affinity for various transporter receptors (muscarinic, histaminic, and norepinephrine). Paroxetine and citalopram have shown, to a greater and lesser extent, a relatively similar affinity for H1 histamine receptors.

Returning to the previous example, it may now be easier to understand why paroxetine and fluoxetine induce almost opposite effects on body weight. Their ability to induce an antidepressant effect would be related to an affinity with the serotonin receptors, while the effects on appetite would be mediated by their respective ability to block (or not) histamine receptors (involved in stimulating appetite). In the light of this example, it is understandable that the indiscriminate substitution of an SSRI with another, on the basis of the "common mechanism of action," is unsustainable. This and other examples should help us to take a first look at the significant differences in widely prescribed drugs due to their efficacy and undisputed tolerability.

The molecules active on the dopamine system are known for reasons totally different from depression. Drugs that act by binding and inhibiting dopamine receptors (antagonists) have been developed as antipsychotics or major tranquilizers; while drugs that act by binding to dopamine receptors by stimulating their action (agonists) are known primarily for their therapeutic action in Parkinson's disease and other movement disorders. The interest in dopamine agonists in the treatment of depressive disorders is a small part of the vast subject of the action of dopaminergic drugs in the central nervous system. In the United States, molecules such as bupropion (Zyban, Wellbutrin) have long been used as antidepressants because of their interesting tolerability profile and the relatively low incidence of manic changes (passage from depression to mania in a patient suffering from bipolar depression) compared to other antidepressants.

Quite curiously, the same drugs or "galenical" preparations (prepared in pharmacies and not produced by companies) have been used in Italy as smoking cessation drugs without any restrictions or need for psychiatric evaluation. The same drugs were used in the United States as antidepressants at the same dosage under specialized psychiatric supervision. Later the situation was resolved and the same drugs were marketed in Italy as prescription antidepressants for the National Health System. We are currently witnessing a growing interest in the application of dopamine-agonist drugs in the treatment of depressive disorders as there are not only data on the efficacy and tolerability of the molecules mentioned above, but also very promising data on the efficacy of the molecules used in Parkinson's disease and in the treatment of resistant depressive forms.

Clomipramine has important anticholinergic, antihistaminic and alpha-adrenergic blocking effects, in addition to considerable arrhythmogenic potential; in doses> 250 mg, follow-up with ECG is recommended. In addition, with these doses, there is a risk of seizures. This is why this drug is usually considered an alternative in the case that SSRIs fail or as an addition to them (although there is no clear evidence that this strategy is effective). It is suggested to avoid the combination of clomipramine and fluvoxamine since the latter inhibits the metabolism of the former, and this is associated with a higher risk of adverse effects. The decision of when to abandon pharmacological treatment should be the presence of adverse effects, the patient's attitudes, comorbidities, the potential for drug interactions, pregnancy or lactation, and other similar factors should be considered.

OCD is frequently a chronic disease and, at times, it is necessary to continue treatment long term; although the remission of moderate or severe cases is rare. In individuals in whom a placebo was administered after clinical remission, a higher recurrence rate was observed, compared to those who continued treatment with escitalopram (52% versus 23%, respectively). In general, there is a consensus that when there is an improvement in symptoms associated with stable medication regimens (and the absence of intolerable adverse effects or other factors), treatment should continue. There is evidence that serotonin and noradrenaline reuptake inhibitors (SNRIs), such as venlafaxine, are effective in treating individuals with refractory SSRI OCD, with response rates of up to 76%. However, in other studies, this drug seems to be inferior to paroxetine; the current tests do not allow us to recommend monotherapy with SNRI to treat OCD.

Recaptation

Reuptake is the process by which 5-HT is removed from the synaptic cleft. The serotonin reuptake sites are located in nerve terminals, especially the CNS, and in several specialized cells such as platelets and enterocytes (Gonzalez-Heydrich and Peroutka, 1990). The SERT transporter, which belongs to the SLC family of solute transporters (Solute Carrier Family) and which is associated with the transport of Na +, Cl- and K + (Blakely et al., 1997), carries out this mechanism of reuptake. The SERT protein has 630 amino acids and has 12 transmembrane domains (Hansen et al., 2011) located on the cell membranes around the synapse or along the axons (Zhou et al., 1998). In the human brain, the density of SERT transporter varies depending on the region, being the area with more transporters the raphe nuclei and the hypothalamus (Kish et al., 2005).

Metabolism

In regard to metabolism, serotonin is subject to two

reactions to facilitate its excretion. The main catabolic pathway is oxidative deamination by monoamine oxidase (MAO) (Molinoff and Axelrod, 1971) giving rise to its main inactive metabolite, 5-hydroxy-indoleacetic acid (5-HIAA). In the digestive system, glucuronidases and other enzymes (Airaksinen et al., 1965) also degrade serotonin. All these enzymes involved in the degradation of serotonin are localized intracellularly, which requires the uptake of serotonin by the cells to proceed to their subsequent inactivation (Fuller and Wong, 1990).

Receptors

The receptors for serotonin are located in the cell membrane R and mediate the effects of the neurotransmitter as an endogenous ligand. There are 7 large types of receptors that, with the exception of the 5-HT3 receptor, a receptor linked to an ion channel, are coupled to the G protein and activate a cascade of intracellular second messengers that will give rise to inhibitory or excitatory responses depending on the receiver (Nichols and Nichols, 2008). The 5-HT2A receptor in particular, whose genetic locus will be the subject of analysis in this work, is a membrane receptor coupled to the G protein that is widely distributed throughout the body (blood vessels, CNS and in the periphery, gastrointestinal tract). In the CNS, it is expressed, above all, in the vicinity of most serotonergic terminal areas. At the peripheral level, it is expressed mainly in platelets and in different types of cells of the cardiovascular system, in fibroblasts, and in neurons of the peripheral nervous system (Chen et al., 1992). The activation of the receptor produces an increase in the release of inositol triphosphate, which in turn promotes the increase of intracellular Ca^{2+} causing excitatory reactions (Nichols and Nichols, 2008).

- Low levels of serotonin in the body can lead to depression, fatigue, negative attitude, irritability, mood swings, anger, insomnia or difficulty falling asleep, memory problems, headache, anxiety symptoms, emotional hypersensitivity, dysthymia, etc.

- Presenting high levels of serotonin can also be harmful. Having too much serotonin in the body can cause Serotonin Syndrome. This syndrome usually appears as a consequence of drug use (ecstasy, amphetamines, etc.) or some antidepressants and analgesics. This chemical is generated in our own body; a unique biochemical conversion process generates it. The cells responsible for producing it use the enzyme tryptophan hydroxylase. Tryptophan, combined with this enzyme, forms 5-hydroxytryptophan, also known as serotonin.

Of the 40 million brain cells, many of them are directly or indirectly influenced by serotonin. This chemical is involved in many health-related processes: appetite and sleep control, mood regulation, activation, mediating sexual arousal, and pain regulation.

- <u>Mood regulation</u>: A mismatch in the production of this substance can have very negative effects on our well-being, on our way of feeling, and behaving. Low levels of serotonin lead us to become angrier, more irritable, to show behaviors that are more impulsive, etc. People with depression tend to have low levels of this substance. In addition, it is believed that the reason why some people are in a bad mood when they wake up, is the descent of this substance at dawn.

- <u>Appetite control</u>: Before an adequate level of serotonin, we feel satiety and we stop eating. If, on the other hand, the levels are low, we feel the need to eat carbohydrates and any caloric food. Too high levels of this substance can also be associated with the appearance of diarrhea; however, an excessive deficit of this substance can cause constipation.

- <u>Regulate the dream</u>: Throughout the day, serotonin levels fluctuate based on our internal clock and circadian rhythm curves. These curves determine the internal schedule that our body follows to know when people have to sleep, eat, etc. Thus, the levels of 5-HT (serotonin receptors) tend to reach their maximum in the sunniest moments of the day, while they go down during deep sleep. The appropriate thing is that there is a balance in their levels, otherwise, it will cause trouble sleeping (insomnia).

- <u>Mediator in sexual desire and libido</u>: Serotonin is directly proportional to sexual desire. High levels of this substance are associated with a lack of libido or sexual desire. While low levels tend to be associated with behaviors aimed at the pursuit of satisfaction of sexual desire. This is because after ejaculating or having an orgasm, the amount of serotonin in the brain increases considerably, which causes a state of pleasure and tranquility. Therefore, excessively high levels of serotonin are associated with a drop in libido, less sexual intercourse, but a higher emotional connection with one's partner.
- <u>Regulation of pain</u>: The brain uses this substance to perpetuate the signs of chronic pain in the local nerves. When local damage occurs, serotonin is released,

producing in our brain a signal of transient and slight pain due to the activation of afferent neurons. This substance is involved in the neuronal signal of pain and also intervenes in chronic pain.

- <u>Serotonin and control of our body temperature</u>: Another function of serotonin is thermal regulation. This substance participates in an important way in the body homeostasis allowing the modulating of core temperature. Although the internal or external factors of our body promote a change in temperature, this substance is responsible for maintaining a thermal regulation to allow the survival of our cells.

- <u>Minimizes levels of aggressiveness</u>: Another function of serotonin is to stabilize our emotional state in situations of stress. This substance helps to inhibit impulsiveness, violent behavior, and aggressiveness. People who frequently exhibit aggressive or violent behavior may have lower levels of serotonin.

Action mechanisms

There are studies that prove that this neurotransmitter can be related to intestinal function. Specialists in that area claim that it regulates intestinal function since serotonin is able to regulate appetite, so the intestine has the ability to digest food at the correct time, which would prevent you from suffering from constipation or flatulence.

Mood and States of Encouragement

Serotonin sends stimuli to the brain that can be evidenced in your moods; it is, where people sometimes inadvertently manifest unwittingly feelings of sadness or happiness. There are diverse opinions in the world that compare serotonin with lethal drugs, and how they wreak havoc on the human body.

Coagulation

This chemical substance helps when you suffer a wound in any part of your body; the platelets that exist in the human body release serotonin, which in turn, sends signals to the brain and to the nervous system, which results in making the blood vessels contract, forming blood clots that begin to heal the wound.

Sickness

Within the favorable functions for the human being, serotonin can increase when a person ingests chemical substances harmful to their health, the speed of the digestive system increases, causing the person to suffer from diarrhea and vomiting, thus expelling that toxic substance.

Bone density

The medical specialists conclude that all excesses in any area of life are not favorable, much less in health; these claim that osteoporosis in humans, in many cases, is due to high levels of serotonin.

Sexuality

It has been shown that people who have high levels of

this neurotransmitter manifest low sexual desire indexes which leads to another series of problems in the life of a couple.

The Hormone of Happiness

Much is said about the relationship that serotonin has with the moods that a person can demonstrate on a normal day; in the same way, they relate to the response that people have to any situation that generates stress. When a person has serotonin levels that are not regular or normal, they can have severe depression and sudden mood swings, anxiety, and in turn, cope by consuming food without control, causing the person to gain weight. Science, in its attempt to find a logical explanation to all the processes that make up the proper functioning of the human body, has determined that serotonin can be generated almost entirely in the digestive system of the human being and the brain, in the same way. It can be found in the central nervous system because its neurotransmitter function is widely proven.

Normal values of this hormone

The medical test used to measure serotonin levels in the blood is called "the serotonin level." It can be identified as a result of normal ranges of 101 to 283 nanograms per milliliter (ng / mL). In order to reach a precise medical diagnosis, many patients go to their doctors in order to find a cure for their suffering - high levels of serotonin can trigger tumors in the liver or digestive system - most people affected at the time of routine examinations have high levels of this substance in both urine and feces.

Several lines of research have supported the importance of serotonin (5-HT) in the pathophysiology of OCD. These include a) Serotonin reuptake inhibitors (SSRIs) have been shown to be the most effective in the treatment of OCD. b) The decrease in the levels of 5-hydroxyindolacetic acid (5-HIAA) in the cerebrospinal fluid has been correlated with clinical response to SSRIs. c) Substances that increase serotonergic transmission, such as L-tryptophan and Lithium, have been successful in reinforcing serotonergic medication in non-responder patients. d) In addition, children with OCD without previous treatment, treated with paroxetine, showed reductions in the volume of the caudate nuclei after successful treatments, a finding that was correlated with clinical improvement.

However, studies with several indirect measures of serotonin in patients with OCD, have produced equivocal findings. It was found that adolescents with OCD had normal platelet levels of 5-HT, compared with healthy volunteers (Flament, 1987), and adults with OCD showed imipramine binding and 5-HT uptake similar to normal control subjects. A cohort composed of adolescents and adults with OCD observed a difference in the binding of imipramine but not in the uptake of 5-HT. In addition, patients who were successfully treated with SSRIs for depression or OCD, experienced tryptophan depletion; while in depressed patients, there was a reappearance of depression, in OCD patients, obsessive compulsive symptoms did not reappear.

Test drugs that are supposedly specific for 5-HT, metaclorofenylpiperazine (MCPP), tryptophan, fenfluramine, and metergoline (an agonist as 5HT specific), have produced contradictory results. MCPP produced elevated temperature and increased obsessive compulsive symptoms according to one study, and it seems that this exacerbation predicts lack of response to SSRIs. Furthermore, when it is administered after three months of treatment with clomipramine, it does not produce an acute accentuation of the symptoms as severe as when the medication is applied to patients without prior treatment. Fenfluramine does not produce an increase in obsessive compulsive symptoms. The metergoline, a specific agonist of 5-HT, diminishes the symptoms only slightly. The lack of response to these agents suggests that there are other relevant transmission systems in OCD. Combination of serotonergic-noradrenergic activity (or effects on calcium channels) has been proposed.

Tryptophan, also known as 5-HTP (5-hydroxytryptophan), is a nutrient found in high-protein foods such as meat, fish, turkey and dairy products. Its importance in psychiatry is because it is the direct precursor of serotonin. Currently, serotonin is closely related to mood disorders or affective disorders, and most antidepressant medications work by increasing the availability of this substance in the space between one neuron and another. Serotonin influences almost all brain functions, including stimulating the GABA (gamma-benzoic acid) system, and although it is only one among hundreds of other neurotransmitters in the brain, currently serotonin is considered one of the most important of these. Serotonin levels determine whether the person is depressed, prone to violence, irritated, impulsive, or greedy.

Just as serotonin can elevate mood and produce a sense of well-being, its lack in the brain or abnormalities in its metabolism has been related to very serious neuropsychic conditions, such as Parkinson's disease, neuromuscular dystonia, Huntington's disease, tremor family, restless legs syndrome, problems with sleep, etc. Psychiatric problems, such as depression, anxiety, aggression, compulsive behavior, affective problems, among others, have also been associated with malfunctioning of the serotonergic system. With this physiological basis, some researchers claim that by increasing the natural precursors of serotonin, one can safely raise their levels and relieve depression, pain, and craving for carbohydrates. Tryptophan, taken as a dietary supplement, may be effective against depression and supplement the action of traditional antidepressants. Tryptophan can be found in high concentrations in the seed of a legume called "Griffonia simplicifolia," found in West Africa. Milk and its derivatives are also sources of 5HTP, as are turkey meat. Other sources of tryptophan: curd, meat, fish, banana, date, peanuts, all foods rich in protein.

Serotonin and Mood

By the middle of this century, medicine began to suspect that there are very likely to be chemicals acting on brain metabolism capable of providing depressive status. This has resulted, in the current knowledge of neurotransmitters and neuroreceptors, very much related to brain activity. In fact, some neurotransmitters, notably serotonin, noradrenaline, and dopamine, are closely associated with the affective state of people. Research that initially sought to support the theory that depression depends (also) for low levels of serotonin, took as its starting point the observation that a tryptophan-free diet, to the point of producing a very low plasma peak of this amino acid, resulted in a moderate depressive state (Charney). Tryptophan, as we saw above, is a natural precursor of serotonin.

Tests have also been performed on severely depressed patients, as well as on suicidal patients, with very low serotonin levels in the spinal fluid of these people. Therefore, it is more acceptable nowadays to believe that the depressed patient is not only a sad person but in fact, it is more certain to believe that the depressed person is a person with a disorder of the affectivity, concomitant or provided by, of neurotransmitters and neuroreceptors. The most typical affective disorder is Depression, with its entire known clinical picture and several other factors which contribute to its cause - among them, the importance of the cerebral biochemistry is emphasized more and more. Anxious pictures such as panic, phobias, somatizations or even generalized anxiety are very frequent affective problems, and it is already accepted that all of them have as their psychic basis, the changes in affectivity.

Antidepressants are drugs that increase psychic tone by improving mood and, consequently, improving one's performance overall. It is believed that the antidepressant effect occurs at the expense of an increased availability of neurotransmitters in the CNS, notably serotonin (5-HT), noradrenaline or norepinephrine (NE) and dopamine (DA). By blocking 5HT2 serotonin receptors, antidepressants also work as anti-migraine drugs. The antidepressant action site, especially the tricyclics, is in the limbic system, increasing norepinephrine and serotonin in the synaptic cleft. This increased availability of the neurotransmitters in the synaptic cleft is achieved by inhibiting the reuptake of these amines by presynaptic receptors. There also appears to be a decrease in the number of pre-synaptic alpha-2 receptors with the use of tricyclic antidepressants, whose feedback stimulation would inhibit the release of noradrenaline. Thus, less of these receptors, plus noradrenaline, would be available in the synaptic cleft. Therefore, two mechanisms related to reuptake: one directly inhibiting reuptake and one decreasing the number of receptors. It is important, in relation to the pharmacokinetics of tricyclic antidepressants, to know the latency period to obtain the therapeutic results.

Serotonin and Serotonergic Systems: Group of Indolamines

There are more than a dozen isolated serotonin receptors divided into 7 major families. Alterations in these neurotransmitters occur in a variety of psychological disorders ranging from a personality disorder, anxiety, depression, eating disorder, schizophrenia, drug-induced psychoses, sensitivity to pain and sleep disorders. There seems to be a relationship between 5HT (serotonin) levels and power. It has been found that in the blood of the dominant male monkey, there is twice as much serotonin as in the dominated monkeys. It seems that an increase in noradrenaline provides a posture opposed to that of dominance: that of submission. In the leader monkey, the elevated 5HT appears to be maintained by the submissive conduct received from its followers. Everything indicates that the same happens between men.

If the leader monkey is removed from the group, its serotonin drops to normal. However, if the leader is removed and, at the same time, the production and release of serotonin is increased in one of the subordinates by supplying him with tryptophan, which is a precursor of serotonin (5HT), plus some medicine that acts as a selective inhibitor of serotonin and reuptake of serotonin (fluoxetine, sertraline, paroxetine and others), the medicated monkey tends to acquire the power that was in the hands of the dominant monkey and thus, the former dominant becomes "any one John." The same event has been demonstrated in lobsters. Among animals, the most powerful and dominant, contrary to popular wisdom, is not the strongest and most aggressive. Among the wolves, the dominant male is often political and builds coalitions to receive cooperation from others in their hunts and in the defense of predators.

There are studies that speculate that women because they are more submissive, present more depressive disorders than men do. The submissive posture of the woman to the man, defended and encouraged by various religions as the correct way for the couple to live, was thought as the main factor in the decrease of serotonin release (as reported in monkeys) and consequently of the onset of depression sadness, apathy, tiredness, various pains, irritability and impulsivity, insomnia, etc.). In addition, low serotonin is associated with impulsivity. This is nothing but a lesser ability and openness to the various possibilities of actions in the face of problems; so is a low dopamine. It was also suggested that a low 5HT would work producing greater sensitivity to rejection. In this condition, described more often among women, one becomes highly vulnerable to non-acceptance or loss. These and other symptoms gave rise to "Borderline Personality

Disorder." These patients usually also have other disorders at the same time, such as Hysterical, Narcissistic and Anti-Social Personality Disorders.

The so-called "borderline" patients, as well as the so-called antisocial, narcissistic, and hysterical, seem to have a common factor: extreme extroversion. If this idea is correct, we can speculate that these emotional and cognitive disorders are associated with the failure of extroverts to make appropriate connections with the desired persons. We can then deduce that it is the failure to achieve connections with these people, rather than the extroversion itself, which must be associated with a decrease in serotonin produced or released in the neuronal synapses of these people. The idea assumes that the normal social environment of every day (especially the relationships between loved ones) continually maintains an appropriate level of serotonin release. Now, if the person is loved and respected by those who matter to her, her 5HT levels tend to get higher and perhaps because of the higher rate of serotonin, make her less outgoing; if that happens, she becomes more introverted than extroverted. Now, thinking the opposite of the above: if the person does not achieve the desired connections, that is, there is rejection, normal levels of serotonin are lowered in the face of failure to keep the social contacts desired. At the same time, there is a tendency for behaviors associated with impulsive aggression, greater sensitivity to rejection, the dread of being alone, and other diverse signs and symptoms described among patients with Borderline Personality Disorder. There is a book about "Borderlines" with an interesting title, which I do not remember exactly, but I remember the message: "I hate you, but I cannot live without you." These patients are hypersensitive to any minimal fact, which are interpreted as rejection. In these cases, if the couple separates, the patient enters in deep despair for the loss; often leaves for the aggression of the spouse and/or to assault himself, such as, for example, attempting suicide.

The above ideas as hypotheses seek to relate social situational factors (loss of important contacts) with important

Effects of Serotonin and Dopamine in Obsessive Compulsive Disorder

biological factors (decreased serotonin release) in behavior control. Conventional wisdom suggests that conduct is under the control of the inborn and learned; sometimes it is one, now the other, the strongest or most powerful. If a poor person has a low level of 5HT, one could argue that their poverty is biologically founded. However, correlation does not prove causality and it is possible that factors associated with poverty, such as lack of power, deprivation (misery, lack of what is necessary for life) of children, poor diet, and social isolation, can contribute to a low level of cerebral serotonin.

4 METHODOLOGY

Introduction

This section defines how the research will be conducted. Within this chapter, it is explained how the sample will be selected, its size, how data will be collected, the research design adopted and target population. According to Savin-Baden and Major (2013, p.23), a complete methodology description needs to highlight how the data was analyzed and prepared for presentation as results. Important to note is that the data analysis procedure depends on the research design and the nature of the information obtained from the respondents or sources. In some instances, data trimming may be necessary.

The relevance of findings and conclusions widely rely on upon quality of the research methods, data collected, mode of analyzing the data, and its presentation. This explains why this section is devoted to the depiction of the techniques and strategies which will be with a particular goal to acquire the information, and the manner through which it will be investigated (Savin-Baden & Major, 2013, p. 94). All these will help in the preparing of the information and the definition of conclusions.

Method and Design

The analysis of the topic would involve carrying out a review of the literature to get views of different authors and researchers regarding the same. In the process of carrying out the study in question, there was the analysis of relevant literature as this provided the opportunity to analyze available scientific articles on the current research relating to the relationship between serotonin and dopamine in OCD patients. The relevant literature provided a wealth of resources that made it easy to address the topical issue under study. The materials that were used in the examination ensure that they were of the right standards. Moreover, the contents of the literature used were analyzed through the right procedures and regarding the right guidelines to confirm their quality. The method used was to help in getting the right interpretation of the study topic. Literature review helped in collecting the necessary data and to help in orienting, assessing and making the right conclusions on the basis of existing evidence.

Quality Review

To get the right quality, the sources that were used conformed to various qualitative analyses; quality control was then done on the books that were used in the literature used for the study. The quality controls were the standards that were used to ensure that the sources used for the analysis conformed to the standards of research. In this way, quality control ensured that there was the proper search of literature used for examination and only the peer-reviewed was employed in the research. Such was done to ensure that all the books used, thereof, confirmed to the topical issue and helped with the required information.

Reliability

Reliability and validity are frequently raised as critical

components of research to support objectivity. According to Wolcott (1995), reliability is an artifact in fieldwork, because the rigor associated with it redirects the attention to the research process rather than the research findings. Obtaining consistency of results with a structured scientific design does not always mean that the results are accurate. Nevertheless, the reliability of findings should be considered in fieldwork, but not to the extent to turn to statistical manipulations to validate our claims.

Ethical Concerns

To ensure that the study was ethical, and upheld the integrity and authenticity of research, there were various standards which helped in providing the right direction and guided researchers in various ways. In this process, the research team ensures that all the data contained in literature used were of high quality and references were very clear. Determination of the available literature was based on three factors: credibility, reliability, and transferability. The main aim of ensuring that the literature was credible was to ascertain that the data from the sources were written in an objective manner and they conformed to the way of thinking of researcher. In this case, the credibility used ensured that the sources contained the required data that reflected the need of patients. Credibility was determined through searching of different databases and brought our similar results and findings. Moreover, credibility ensured that data from the sources were both scientific and provided reliable and high-quality data. Reliability, on the other hand, ensured that the data contained in the sources could stand the test of time, and that result could last for a long time. Finally, the aspect of transferability of the sources was an important aspect of choosing the sources in that it ensured that the sources selected for the study related to other findings in the same field.

There was an objective review of all findings used in the study as all sources used in the study were required to conform to the required standards. Literature that did not conform to the standards was excluded to ascertain that there was uniform quality in the doing of the research. By using very many different

Effects of Serotonin and Dopamine in Obsessive Compulsive Disorder sources, there was credibility in the information of the research process.

Ethical Considerations

Because the research employed the use of literature from other research works, it was apparent that the research was ethical. There was also protection of the research process and this helped in ascertaining that researchers did not tamper with primary data and that there was not tamper with the final outcome of the research. There were various quality checks of the research process.

This study will not be considered unethical or controversial as it is based on research and previously conducted studies that have been researched ethically, tested and approved. According to Polit and Beck (2013), a researcher can consciously or unconsciously influence the result by distorting content and meaning in previous research. One aspect of the processing of the data is the scientific terminology and the English language. Carefulness will be observed in the interpretation and translation of the articles. In the event of difficulties with the translation, a dictionary and a third party with will be used. The study included articles with varying forms of results. To actively exclude results that were emissive to other included research, leads to a confusion of the current knowledge situation.

5 COMPILATION OF FINDINGS

European diagnostic tradition considers Obsessive Compulsive Disorder (O.C.D), as an independent nosological entity. The presence of anxiety symptoms does not imply including OCD within anxiety disorders because they are frequently associated, but not invariably to OCD, and are considered secondary to it. The American psychiatry regards it as an anxiety disorder. In the classification DSM-1I, the concept of obsessive compulsive neurosis is accepted and in the DSM-III, it is included within the Anxiety disorder; the DSM-IV draft seems to continue in this line. The Consideration of OCD as an anxiety disorder it has no empirical basis; the obsessions are defined as repetitive, intrusive thoughts that provoke a marked anxiety, and compulsions are repetition behaviors of rituals performed in order to reduce anxiety or prevent it. However, based on the evidence of clinical observation, response to treatment and biological studies makes it be considered OCD as an independent entity with its own evolution. A big number of Neurological disorders have symptoms similar to the compulsive behavior of OCD and this allows us to speculate the possible existence of a neurological basis in this disorder.

Another part has found an increased incidence of minor neurological symptoms in OCD (Denckle, 1988); there is also a relationship between perinatal traumas (Capstick and Saldrup, 1977) and this disorder. There is a strong relationship between OCD and the disorders related to alterations in which the base of the ganglia plays an important role, for example in Parkinson's Post-Encephalitic, in which there is an alteration of said ganglia and it appears with characters like compulsive motor tics and other behaviors. Along with this, a higher association has found, what would be observed due to chance, a connection between OCD and Gilles's syndrome of Tourette. Many of the patients with OCD suffer from marked psychic symptoms of anxiety as somatics, and up to 60% of them suffer from panic attacks. However, these symptoms do not appear in all patients and their presence is not enough to include OCD within the anxiety disorder. Depressive

Effects of Serotonin and Dopamine in Obsessive Compulsive Disorder symptoms are very common in OCD; almost one-third DSM-III-r criteria for major depression (Rasmussen and Bisen, 1992). All this shows is that OCD is a disorder with a very high comorbidity.

    Lopez-Ibor Alino described in 1968: the positive action of clomipramine (CMI) in the then called "obsessional neuroses." The one that this antidepressant, and not others such as imipramine, desipramine or amitriptyline, has, is this profile characteristic which was attributed by Yayuria-Tobias to that the CMI has, compared to others tricyclic antidepressants, a more potent action on serotonin reuptake than on other neurotransmitters such as noradrenaline and serotonin. Subsequent therapeutic studies tend to confirm this hypothesis. Lopez-Thor Alino found that the best predictor of positive response to the CMI is its administration intravenously, which bypassing the effect of the first passage through the liver, allows plasma concentrations of CMI compared to its demethylated metabolite (DM-CMI). Indeed, Mavassakalian (1989) has been able to correlate positively the response to treatment with the

CMI plasma concentration and negatively with the DM- CMI.

Therapeutic experience suggests that serotonergic mechanisms play an important role in obsessive compulsive disorders. However, neurochemical studies have received comparatively less attention than those carried out in other disorders, such as mood disorders in general and depressions in particular. In all of them, the studies are concordant. Depressions, especially major forms or melancholic, suicide attempts, especially violent ones, and suicidal behaviors, are characterized by serotonergic deficits. However, two teams of workers have found a key to unravel the problem: One (Insel, Zohar, Murphy, 1988) has described serotonin activation symptoms after administration of m-CPP, metabolite of trazodone used as a probe serotonergic. Another, that of Lopez-Ibor Alino (1991), who has found an exaggerated answer to another serotonergic probe: the CMI, in obsessive compulsive disorders, has contracted the presence of depressive symptoms. It is possible that there are symptoms of hyper-response to serotonin stimuli in obsessive patients that would be masked when there is a depression associated with Obsessive Compulsive Disorder.

In the most recent papers presented related to this disorder, the most important used neuroimaging and found that structures of the orbito-frontal cortex and the head of the caudate nucleus are affected. Studies of brain biochemical function using positron emission techniques (PET) suggest that patients with this disorder have high metabolism rates in the gyrus orbitalis and in the caudate nucleus although its significance is not yet clear (Baxter et al., 1988, Garter et al., 1989). Possibly these structures constitute a functional circuit in the diverse neurotransmission systems: 5-HT, dopamine, and GABA.

Terminology

In Germany and France was where the in-depth study of psychopathology began and clinical of obsessive pictures. The technical meaning of terms like "obsession," "compulsion," "imperative idea," "mental harassment," "impulse," and "contrary act" did not acquire true development until the last period of the nineteenth century. Previously these terms had been used in ordinary language to refer to mental acts in relation to the will. The word "scruple" ('small, pointed or pointed stone') (Lewis and Short, 1879) was also used in the seventeenth century to refer to repetitive thoughts of a religious nature. The psychiatric terminology of the nineteenth century had three origins: terms inherited from the Greek and Roman periods (for example mania, melancholy, paranoia); language words vulgar with technical meaning (for example hallucination, obsession, stupor); and neologisms (for example lypemania or monomania).

Regarding obsessive disorders, Krafft-Ebing coined, in 1867, the term "Zwansgvorstellung" to refer to irresistible (obsessive) thoughts (Krafft-Ebing, 1879). "Zwang" comes from the high German term "Twang." During the Middle German period, it meant "forcing or oppressing," the root being the word "tvanzkti" (the strip of oneself) from Sanskrit (Monterrat-Esteve, 1971). In 1887, Westphal used that term, rigorizing the concept of the 'forced' (obsessive) and that as Kurt Schneider (1975) highlights, it constituted the "starting point of the whole doctrine of obsessions". Westphal (1877) equated representations to ideas and suggested that obsessive states they had a disorder of intellectual function; this intellectualist interpretation exercised a very remarkable influence. This author established a distinction between presentations as acts mental illnesses (obsessive ideas or ruminations) and as indicators of action (compulsions).

Terms like "Zwangshandlung," "Zwangsphanomenen" and "Zwangszustand" were coined later to refer to iterative actions (Montserrat-Esteve, 1971a). "Zwang" is applicable to both thoughts and obsessive acts, and this ambiguity is of historical interest. "Zwangsvorstellung" was translated as an *obsession* in Britain and as a *compulsion* in the United States; as a compromised solution, the obsessive disorder finally emerged (Rado, 1959). Griesinger (1868) introduced a second root word, "Schut," which means "disease or passion" (Montserrat-Esteve, 1971a), "mania" (Soria, 1959) or better "cachexia" (López Ibor,

1960). The compound term "Grubelnsucht" corresponds to the ruminative disease of Griesinger. Grubeln is an old German term that is equivalent to 'racking your brains'. Donath (1897), at a conference given at the Royal Medical Society of Budapest, in November 1895, proposed the term "anancasmus" to name the picture that Thomsen (1895) had called "idiopathic obsessive state." He did derive it from the Greek "anaké" that means "destiny, fatality." This third terminological root was used especially for adjectival and so, Schneider (1950) coined the derivative "anankastic personality (WHO, 1978)."

Donath created what he wanted to designate idiopathic "obsessive" states; which for him, constituted a defined clinical unit from which the phobias of the "neurasthenia". However, several authors, both national and foreign, use the term "anancasmo" to designate indistinctly obsessions and phobias (Montserrat-Esteve, 197 1a). In German, there are several terms to designate drives and related phenomena. In "Etudes P.sychiatriques," volume II, gathers the main ones and gives the

Effects of Serotonin and Dopamine in Obsessive Compulsive Disorder

French translation: Antrieb, Impuis, Einfall, Trieb, Drang, Suc / it and Zwang that respectively translates by: 'incidence', 'Drive', 'crisis', 'instinct', 'drive', 'need' and 'obsession'. Lopez Ibor (1967a), in his article entitled "¿Instintos o puliones?," echoed the discussion around the translation of the word "Trieb" in the wake of Lacan's publications on the Freudianism, (cited by Lopez Ibor, 1967a) "in Freud, the distinction between instinct and drive."

In England, it was translated by instinct. The other country, from which the original knowledge of the obsessive subjects starts, is France. In the French language, they were using different names to name the obsessive states: man/e sons délíre (Pinel, 1889), matad/e dii doute (Falret, 1866), folle dii doute ayec délire by toucher (Legrand du Saulle, 1875), folie hucide (Trelat, 1861), délire emotzf (Morel, 1866), onomatomania (Charcot and Magnan, 1885, Seglas, 1891). Esquirol isolates monomania as a delirium limited to a single subject or a number of them, with excitement and predominance of a joyful and expansive passion (1838). Apart from "amenomania" or "mania," properly said, which is equivalent to the current mania, and the "lipemania" (of Greek lypé, 'sadness') which corresponds to the melancholy of today, most of the monomanias designated the current obsessions and impulses. The number of monomanias proliferated and the reaction was not made to wait. Pi Molist (1864) accepted the term, but opposed his hypertrophy, and yet it said: "from old-time dates the custom of manias certain skinny, whims and particular tastes rooted in some men, and this tenor has admitted the use of the voices "melomanía," "metromanía," "bibliomanía," and others, but until recently, no one had bristled at the idea of turning the passionate into a madman exceedingly for music, poetry or books" (Montserrat-Esteve, 1971).

Even then, the different meanings of the word *mania* gave rise to confusion between the psychiatrists who investigated her. In fact, today it still has different meanings: a) exaggerated hobby, b) obsessive disorder (arithmomania) and c) opposite phase to melancholy in the manic-depressive psychosis. Although the corresponding adjectives highlight, in part, these differences; so in the first and second case, we talk about "maniacs" and in the third of "Maniacs Monomania," was a version of the concept of insanity or partial madness. Before the nineteenth century and during this, this category was differentiated from insanity or general madness in four basic aspects: a) intensity of symptoms, b) degree of involvement of the personality, c) deterioration of selective psychological functions and d) exclusivity of delirium (Berrios, 1981; Kageyama, 1984). The third criterion was made possible thanks to the reintroduction at the beginning of this century of the pathology of the faculties; that is, the perspective that the human mind can be analyzed operationally in faculties. This was greatly influenced by Kant and the Scottish philosophers (A Brecht,1970; Brooks, 1976; Hilgard, 1980; Berrios, 1984).

The term *obsession* did not really acquire current medical use in France until the decade 1880-1890. It was from Luys (1883) and Falret (1889) when it acquired his clinical concept, which was rigorized thanks to the works of Morel and Falret. Luys (1883), referred as "obsessions pathologies" to all those subjective events which are anomalous and repetitive without an external source. Until then, the term had served to describe the action of an external abstract agent that harassed the individual (Littre, 1877). Luys represents, then, a great innovation when converting obsessions into something internal; this was well accepted (Falret, 1889, Bail, 1892). Magnan included obsessions among psychic "stigmates des dégénérés."

At that time, Italian authors also involved obsessions with psychoses and they spoke of rudimentary paranoia (Morselli), of diathesis of incoercibilidad (Tanzi), of incoercibles ideas (Tamburini) or of fixed ideas (Buccola, 1880). In the English language, the terminological evolution followed similar paths (Berrios, 1977). From the sixteenth century, "obsession" was used to describe the act of being besieged by the devil. Tuke (1894) referred to imperative ideas and Miclde (1896) to mental harassment. In the Nomencíator of Diseases, prepared in London by the Committee of the Royal College of Physicians, an obsessive insanity was included (Royal College of Physicians, 1906). The

Effects of Serotonin and Dopamine in Obsessive Compulsive Disorder

term obsession was introduced in the main medical journals of the time (Editorial, 1901; Leader, 1904). Shan (1904) publishes a review of these disorders, using the "obsession" word. The term also appears in American literature around the same period (Diller, 1902).

In general terms, while the German authors describe the obsessions in terms extracted from the common language, they also tended to consider them as a functional disorder. The French, using a terminology with a psychiatric background, were more predisposed to interpret those as psychotic or psychopathic. While for Freud, the center of gravity of his "obsessive neurosis," was rooted in its psychological determinants, as well as for Adíer or for Steckel with his "Anancastic parapathy", in Janet, the constitutional, the "psychasthenic" was essential. From these differences, the German authors of the last century studied more forcefully *symptoms*, more than *obsessives*, who as such were ubiquitous. On the other hand, drive comes from the Latin impulses, 'action and effect of impeler'. At the same time, impeler comes from the Latin impelere, 'to give push, to incite, to stimulate', already classically defined as the necessary action for the internal phenomenon of appetite to be translated into action. Compulsion comes from the Latin compulsium, and derived from compulsium is supine from compettere, 'Action and effect of compeler', which in turn derives from compeliere and is equivalent to "forcing a person to act against their will, from their natural impulses" (Montserrat-Esteve, 1971).

Due to the North American influence and especially of the Spanish-speaking countries, compulsion is no longer taken in the wrong sense of impulse, but, has been assigned another equivalent to "Zwang" or "anancasmo" and, therefore, covers all of the obsessive phenomena (thoughts, memories, forgetfulness, occurrences, feelings, acts, etc.).

Obsessive disorders in the nineteenth century

The first clinical descriptions of obsessive patients are attributed to the parents of the French psychiatry. The current sense of *obsession* is that of an "idea, image or word that imposes the spirit in a repeated and incoercible way" dating from 1799 with Wartburg (Berrios, 1986). Westphal (1877) defines obsessions as "parasitic ideas, which, by remaining intact the intelligence and without there being an emotional or passionate state, arise before the conscience, imposing on her against her will, going through and preventing the game normal of ideas and being, always recognized by the patient as abnormal; you miss yourself." Here, part of the intellectual pathogenic assumption of obsessions and obsessive beliefs are not always recognized as strange by the sick, and the effective components that must enter, in their own right, into a definition who wants to be universal (Costa Molinari, 1971a).

For Westphal, the following are essential characteristics of the obsessions:

1) There is always an awareness of the illness.
2) They have a character of irrepressibility.
3) They occur in subjects with intact intelligence.

For Schneider (1942), "obsessions are contents of conscience that manifest themselves with the subjective experience of compulsion, of not being able to be avoided, even though in conditions of relative calm, can be judged as absurd or unmotivated dominant." This definition involves a germ of confusion among overvalued ideas and the obsessive ones, as Lopez Ibor (1966) has pointed out, even within the obsessive domain a wide range of phenomena that can be qualified as contents of conscience.

For Bumke (1924) obsessions are "representations whose immovability, also felt by the patient, can be sufficiently explained by the action of pathological causes that normally determine the persistence of representations in consciousness (state of mood, affective tone of the same, inability to reach a conclusion) to which could be added, for certain cases, and whose content the patient himself comes to judge as logically false when you examine it under conditions of tranquility." With his definition breaks the classical conception for most authors, for whom the essential aspect of the obsession would be its strange, absurd and parasitic character, and tries to differentiate them from hypochondriacal and overvalued ideas, as well as from slime phenomena post-encephalic.

Friedmann (1907) is, along with Westphal, another of the leading figures in the delimitation of the concepts about obsessive pathology. Together, they define the "Zwangsvorstelhung" as "those representations of doubt, concern, and waiting, by which by their nature remain incapable of logical finishing and whose property is to force its carrier against its will, already through a nervous excitement strongly increased, and already through primary inhibitions of thought and decision." This distinguishes three groups: a) depressive ideas, b) affective reactions and c) fears and doubts of different kinds. Since a genetic point of view differentiates, overvalued ideas heavily loaded from an effect of the weakly colored. In the first belong the depressive ideas, the anguish, really conditioned by the wait and, in part, the scruples. The second belongs to phobias, including shyness and fear of being observed, hypochondriac ideas and, in a characteristic way, "neurotic" effective ideas.

Esquirol (1838) classified the obsessive phenomena of Mademoiselle F. as a form of monomanía (délire partid), thus inaugurating the line that considered obsessive disorders as a kind of insanity or madness. This author defined monomania as "a chronicle disease of the brain without fever, characterized by a partial lesion of the intellect, emotions or the will" (Rachman and Hodson, 1980). Esquirol observed that Mademoiselle F. described her thoughts as irresistible and that seemed to have introspection about his symptoms, which made him think that irresistibility was the manifestation of a secondary disturbance of the volitional faculty (Billod, 1847).

In the second half of the nineteenth century, while in Germany there was talk of "representations" and forced "acts" without prejudging its nature, in France qualified the obsessions of crazy things. French authors cataloged the obsessions between delusions. So Morel described the obsessive paintings under the title of "délire émot" (1866), but this delirium did not mean what today it is usually understood as such! Morel considered it "not as a psychosis, but as a neurosis, as a special disease of affectivity "(Pitres and Regis, 1902). Morel's emphasis on the emotional aspects of the disorder represented a clear innovation with respect to previous intellectualist interpretations. It explained the "impulse psychomotor "that leads to compulsion as an "exalted affective state." Baruk (1959) called this emotional dimension the "infernal circle of obsession" and pointed out that it was precisely for this reason why Morel had called it "emotive delirium". The clinical description described by Morel was very similar to Janet's psychasthenia (1903). Morel considered this constellation of symptoms as a neurosis and of the "functional injury;" at this time, this was imputed to the autonomous system (Lopez Pinero, 1983). He underlined the perspective vegetative nervous. This reclassification of Morel was accepted in French psychiatry for two reasons: fundamental, first, as it proposed an alternative to the German vision that obsessive states were a thought disorder similar to paranoia (Meyer, 1906), and secondly, it allowed a rational classification of various somatic symptoms, considered today as "anxious equivalents" (Doyen, 1885). Luys (1883) followed and developed Morel's hypothesis, for *emotions* and *actions* had separate cortical localization, and *nervous* could, depending on the area affected, give rise to strange ideas, or compulsive acts.

Luys divides the obsessions into three groups: those that remain predominantly in the intellectual domain, those that fall within the sphere of feelings (and here includes anxious melancholy and some emotional delusions) and those that appear above all in the psychomotor domain and lead to the performance of extravagant acts, automatic and impulsive. Some French authors, including Falret (1889), include in the concept of obsessive all the phobic manifestations. The set of obsessions possess the following properties:

1) the sick are aware of their condition,
2) it is frequently observed that they are hereditary,

3) the disease shows a periodic, intermittent character,

4) these morbid states greatly affect all psychic life in the form of anguish, doubt, inability to finish and create disturbances in the affective sphere,

5) they are never accompanied by hallucinations,

6) they never evolve towards them,

7) they never end in dementia, and,

8) they are rarely accompanied by delusional persecutory ideas or melancholy.

Pitres and Regis (1902) defined obsessions as "a morbid syndrome characterized by the anxious experience of parasitic thoughts and emotions that force the subject, and lead to a form of psychic dissociation, whose final state is an unfolding of the conscious personality." These authors divided the obsessive disorders into phobic and ideations, and each of them in diffuse and specific. For Pitres and Regis, the characteristics of obsession were:

1) They often manifest in predisposed subjects.

2) They always belong to the group of emotions of a depressive hue.

3) They are conscious phenomena in the sense that the sick realize the modifications that print their way of being, their character and affectivity.

4) They are involuntary and incoercibles, and the subject is unable to provoke or avoid.

5) They are accompanied by physiological concomitants, strong emotions of type distressing.

6) As a general rule, they do not modify the general mechanism of intelligence.

Thomson (1895) represents it as the forced sensations of bodily and psychic nature, to include movements, acts, language disorders, impulses and forced inhibitions. Even when your criterion tends to encompass a large number of manifestations within the same concept of "obsession," it excludes perversions and phobias (cited by Montserrat-Esteve, 1971). Mickei (1896) states that obsession disorders are mixed with thinking, feeling

Effects of Serotonin and Dopamine in Obsessive Compulsive Disorder and wanting.

Haskovec (1900) distinguishes between the obsessions with 4 groups:

1) genuine fixed ideas in the sense of Griesinger or Westphal,
2) transient and curable states, which often appear in the form of phobias or forced representations that occur in individuals with neuropathic defects and yet, in normal people, under certain external circumstances,
3) forced symptomatic representations and phobias that are manifestations symptoms of neurosis, neurasthenia, hysteria, epilepsy, Basedow's disease and affections of the sympathetic or intoxications, and
4) prodromes of psychosis-melancholy, paranoia, general paralysis, in the case of true forced representations and not delirious ideas.

The first English descriptions of the obsessive syndrome were related to melancholy or depression. They also referred to the concern about religious issues. The terms *scruples* and *religious melancholy* were used to describe this affliction when guilt was the predominant symptom (Hunterland and Mac Alpine, 1963; Insel, 1990a). The controversy held between the supporters of the intellectual or emotional pathogenesis of the obsessions is surpassed by the contribution of Janet that centers the origin of the obsessions, like most psychopathological phenomena, in the decrease of "tension psychological." Up to here, the obsessions had been kept within a semiological framework isolated; it is only from the hand of Janet and Freud that they become part of the neurosis. Janet (1903), in her works, introduces the concept of "psychasthenia." Janet considered obsessive disorders (1903) as a dislocation of function. There was, according to her, a dullness of the mind without anatomical substrate. The obsessions were the concomitant subjective or experience of a feeling of incompleteness that derived from a deep flaw in the "function of the real."

Janet created the category, "psychasthenia" that she extracted from neurasthenia and that contained, among others, obsessive disorders in her work, "L'automatismepsychologique" (1898). Janet considered obsessions as a kind of fixed ideas, which together with hallucinations, constituted "the simple and rudimentary forms of mental activity" (Janet, 1903). Janet encompasses both the French and Spanish concepts of *obsession* and *phobia*. However, there are many authors who do not establish differences between obsession and phobia, in both countries, and even, before and now. For Janet, in her *psychestenia,* it encompasses the disposition of anguish, for phobia and obsession, but later it establishes distinctions. The obsessions are derived directly from feelings of incompleteness and failure of action, while phobias arise from fear of action. For Pitres and Regis, obsession is often nothing more than the exaggerated or intellectualized form of the phobia.

Janet's definition of psychasthenia was etiological and did not propose diagnostic criteria; it was based on theoretical mechanisms such as the reduction of psychological tension and the non-introspective process of incompleteness. Janet's psychological perspective firmly placed the obsessive states in the new territory of the neuroses, which at that time included neurasthenia, hysteria, and psychostenia (López Piñero, 1983). Marchais (1964), according to Janet, defines obsession as "ideological elements or incoercible images that invade the conscious thought and that have a painful character for the anguish that accompanies them; This forces the patient to fight against this parasitism of the thought that judges absurd." For Marchais, the fundamentals of obsessions are the following aspects:

1) The obsessive anguish is constant and does not give place to rest.
2) The thought suffers a parasitism that, without affecting the judgment that remains intact, it acquires an aspect of intrusion and of being strange.
3) A fight is established against this parasitism that gives rise to rituals and obsessive ceremonies.

With Freud, obsessive phenomena become a well-differentiated nosological group within the neuroses. For this author, it is a condition in which the patient does not/cannot discard his absurd ideas and, even if he wants to, he cannot do anything to improve your state. You can only displace or replace your obsession by replacing an absurd idea by another. In these patients, the oppositions that fill the psychic life are particularly accentuated. It highlights the state of doubt that causes in the subject a perpetual indecision. Freud (1895) proposed separating obsessions and phobias, claiming that "in the true obsessions, it is clear that the emotional state is the main element, since it remains unmodified, while the idea associated with it varies." He considered that the reason for this substitution was a defensive reaction (Abwehr) of the ego against an intolerable idea (Freud, 1909).

A year later, he extended his sexual theory of hysteria to obsessions; detection of guilt in the patient indicated or suggested the presence of guilt fronts hidden enjoyment. Freud's conception of obsessions changed at the same time, as his theory of neuroses. The emphasis was going to be put on the structure of the obsessive personality rather than in the mechanical production of obsessive symptoms (Laplanche and Pontalis, 1983). According to the objectivist and descriptive approach, initiated by Pollit (1957) and adopted by several Anglo-Saxon and Scandinavian authors, the obsessive paintings would be: "thoughts, images, feelings, impulses, recurrent or persistent movements that are accompanied by an immediate feeling of subjective compulsion and the desire to oppose them; the fact is recognized by the patient as alien to his personality, even when he has the perception of the nature of it since such symptoms occur in reactions other than the obsessive states. We will define obsessive states as diseases in which obsessions are the predominant characteristics and of which no other disease, organic or psychological, is responsible" (Pollit, 1957). Without a clear definition, "etiopathogenic," aims to describe the reality of the obsessive pictures focusing his natural history.

For Salzman (1981), the fundamental features of obsessions

Effects of Serotonin and Dopamine in Obsessive Compulsive Disorder are:

1) Behavior and thinking persist beyond the need the patient's will,
2) Patients have an extensive variability of phenomena consequence of the strange nature of thoughts, and
3) Still against anxious, the consciousness of the illogical and irrational nature of thought or of the action.

For Oreen (1965):

1) Obsessions manifest in highly intelligent subjects who are clear and conscience.
2) The figure of the obsessive manifestations constitutes representations or other processes.
3) In the field of a series of ideas, effective connotations are always of nature, unpleasant or painful.
4) The "I" declares the contents as foreign and strange.
5) Anxiety is present especially in the forms closest to phobias.

6) The subject sets in motion his defenses that progressively acquire character that is obsessive

7) The obsessive system tends to spread, and

8) The periods of clinical silence are periods of evolution at a low tone.

For Lopez Ibor (1966), "the primary character of obsession is its strangeness and lack of sense. They have, on the other hand, a peculiar dialectical structure, according to which obsession that is born of the self, which cannot control, possess a special coercive characteristic, and are developed only on elements of psychic life susceptible of being directed; they are incoercible and present, and they display a peculiar tendency to the repetition with inability to finish." Ultimately, he considers obsessions as experiences that differ quantitatively from the normal ones and settle in a base in which the essential is the anguish.

History of OCD Classifications

Currently OCD is sometimes framed within anxiety disorders, starting from the psychodynamic approach of Freud;

this is reflected in the Manual Diagnostic and Statistical of the American Psychiatric Association in its first edition (D.S.M.-I) (APA, 1952); D.S.M.-II (APA, 1968) and in the 9th edition of the Classification International of Diseases, of the World Health Organization (I.C.D.-9) (WHO, 1987). However, certain clinical observations that arose in the 1960s raise, for the first time, the possibility that this supposedly unitary building is constituted in reality by clinical pictures that offer deep differences and different causality. In the D.S.M.-III (APA, 1980), the order of distress disorders is reconsidered from radically different conceptual bases. In this new approach, the term, neurosis, is abandoned, implying sharing a common cause. Unconscious conflict leads to inadequate defense mechanisms, resulting in the generation of symptoms. Instead of a supposed etiology, D, S.M.-III bases the classification on the presence of symptoms that are common. A multi-axis system is also established to separately evaluate the personality disorders, organic etiologies, environmental stressors and level of adaptation.

Epidemiology of obsessive compulsive disorders

The presence of recurrent and annoying thoughts (obsessions) or repetitive behaviors, relatively stereotyped, which the individual feels forced to perform (compulsions), but that recognizes as irrational or exaggerated, has been known throughout history like: scruples, religious melancholy, madness of doubt, obsessive neurosis, disease obsessive and more recently, as an obsessive compulsive disorder (APA, 1987). If considered during the 19th century as a form of psychosis, it was included in what is defined psychodynamically as neurosis. This new identity, in some way, has delayed this investigation. The ineffectiveness of psychotherapeutic approaches on the one hand, and advances obtained through biological treatments on another, have boosted their research in line with the search for organic factors to explain their etiology.

Obsessive compulsive disorder was considered a rare disease and with a very poor prognosis (Rasmussen and Tsuang, 1984). Until then, the estimated epidemiological studies were

Effects of Serotonin and Dopamine in Obsessive Compulsive Disorder based on retrospective studies in hospitalized patients. The investigations had important methodological problems due to the lack of structured interviews and homogeneous diagnostic criteria. Rildin, in 1953, estimated that the prevalence of this disorder was five out of every thousand inhabitants, although most researchers suspected that the disorder was more frequent in the general population than what initial studies indicated. It was intuited that given the characteristics of the disease in which the patient is aware of what happens, he fears being "going crazy" and, therefore, being stigmatized, and delays commenting on his symptoms to doctors and even to their own relatives; in some cases until the incapacitation caused by the disorder, prevents him from holding more. An average of 7.5 years, according to different authors, between the onset of symptoms and the request for medical help (Olivares and Vallejo, 1987).

In 1984, the first results of a large-scale epidemiological study were obtained in the USA (Mayers et al., 1984; Robins et al., 1984), showing some results 50 to 100 times higher than what

Rildin estimated in 1953. The initial data, based on approximately 10,000 inhabitants, estimated that 2.5% of the population studied had a history of obsessive compulsive symptoms in his life, enough to meet the DSM-III diagnostic criteria for obsessive compulsive disorder (APA, 1980), and that 1.6% had had the disorder in the six months prior to the interview. If this data was correct, OCD would be the fourth most frequent psychiatric disorder, after phobias, substance abuse, and major depressive disorder! Its prevalence in this study was twice as high as schizophrenia or panic attacks. The final analysis of the data was obtained in 1988 and was consistent with the original data published in 1984 (Karno et al., 1988). This data was subsequently validated by an epidemiological study of 3,258 Edmonton residents in the United States carried out by Blanc et al. in 1988; it obtained a prevalence of 3% and 1.6% in the previous six months. Several authors have criticized these results, on the one hand for having been conducted the interview by non-specialized personnel, and on the other hand, commenting that it had included patients with minimal social or occupational disability secondary to symptoms.

Flament et al., in 1988, in a rigorous study using the same inclusion criteria, estimates the prevalence of obsessive compulsive disorder in the general population between 1% and 2%. They used Leyton's obsession questionnaire on a sample of 5,108 students. Flament established a cut-off point in the severity of the symptomatology; those students who had high scores were again evaluated, this time, by a specialist in psychiatry, to confirm the presence or absence of OCD. The data of this study were extrapolated to the general population. This increase has been reflected in the change of the comment of the DSM-III (APA, 1980) where it says "the disorder is apparently rare in the general population" to "forms mild disorders, may be relatively frequent "in the DSM-III-r (APA, 1987). In 1993, Degonda published a longitudinal study in which a cohort of subjects studied young Swiss adults; the follow-up period was eleven years. The prevalence rate at thirty years old for OCD was 5.5%. The average

age of onset of the disorder was 17.1 (+1/- 4.9 years) for males and 19.1 (+ 1/-l) for females. Degonda also found associations between OCD with all forms of depression, and with others anxiety disorders such as social phobia and agoraphobia. In addition, they found that there was a certain stability in the symptomatology, what these authors interpret, as "patients with OCD, learn to live with their symptoms, without suffering."

Reinzherz et al (1993), in a population of 386 white adolescents, found that lifetime prevalence rates for alcohol consumption/dependence were 34.5%, phobias presented a rate of 22%, drug abuse of 9.4%, major depression of a 9.4%, and post-traumatic stress disorder was 6%, while OCD was 2.1%. Rasmussen et al (1985) found that patients with chronic OCD with compulsions of hand washing are often seen by specialists in dermatology. From a series of 22 cases, only 8 were referred to the psychiatrist. What this author suggests is that dermatologists are able to diagnose anxiety and depression disorders, but that the obsessive compulsive disorder is rarely recognized. Yet, OCD affects both sexes with the same frequency. The data of the literature suggests that a third of the cases start around the age of fifteen, and most do before twenty (Rasmussen et al.); citing 19.8 years as the average age of onset, with a deviation of 9.6 years. Rapoport (1992) publishes a case in which the age of appearance was 2 years old. During childhood and puberty, it is more frequent that OCD is developed in males, while in women usually appearing or getting worse during pregnancy or menstruation.

In geriatric ages, organic factors are the most frequent cause of obsessive compulsive symptoms. On the other hand, Neziroglu et al (1992) evaluated a group of women with obsessive compulsive disorder in which 39% developed symptoms during pregnancy. However, it is still not clear why, during pregnancy, this disorder surfaces. Others seem to present complaints because they do not like the depression that appears in the postpartum period. These authors did not note that pregnancy (in these women) was a situation especially stressful. It is known that steroid hormones exert an influence on the serotoninergic system. Perhaps during pregnancy, changes in this system can determine the appearance of OCD. In different studies, it has been proven possible to verify how estrogens increase synthesis and activity in the dorsal raphe nuclei, while progesterone decreases the hypothalamic accumulation of serotonin. It has also been possible to demonstrate an increase in 5-HT platelets during the first trimester of pregnancy. Schatzberg (1993) postulates the hypothesis that hormonal changes during and after pregnancy produce changes in aminergic function, which are determinants of variations in behavior. Increased secretion of gonadal steroids during pregnancy would be associated with an increase in the obsessive compulsive disorder, while the decrease of estrogen in the postpartum would be associated with an increase in the incidence of depression.

On the contrary, Sichel et al (1993) believed that puerperium (a period of about six weeks post-partum) can be a risk factor to develop an obsessive compulsive pathology. They studied a group of fifteen pregnant women who developed

Effects of Serotonin and Dopamine in Obsessive Compulsive Disorder

obsessive compulsive symptoms during the puerperium, they all met criteria DSM-III-r for OCD. Almost all had intrusive thoughts of doing harm to their children, none had obsessive rituals, yet they subsequently developed a secondary depression, and all presented an excellent response to treatment with selective inhibitors of serotonin reuptake. OCD is a disease of chronic course. Your symptoms show exacerbations and mutations. It can worsen acutely, but the most normal presentation is that the symptoms appear in a subacute course. Unfortunately, the degree of disability that this disease produces is very high. New research techniques allow a better understanding of the basics of neuropsychological aspects of this disease. Currently, it can be diagnosed easily and there are also effective therapies that allow most patients to recover from this terrible disease, or at least survive through a remission or maintenance of it. Karno said in 1988, "... There is evidence that obsessive compulsive disorder is a common mental illness, like other stigmatized and hidden disorders in the past, but it demands a large-scale treatment."

OCD serotoninergic hypothesis

Although a single neurotransmitter system is unlikely to explain the full complexity of OCD, recent efforts to elucidate its pathophysiology have focused primarily on the role of the neurotransmitter 5-hydroxytryptamine (5-HT). The serotonergic hypothesis of OCD, which states that this disorder is linked to serotonin dysfunction, derives mainly from studies on pharmacological treatments. It has been known for more than 35 years that clomipramine (Anafranil), a potent serotonin reuptake inhibitor, is effective in reducing OCD symptoms. Since then, numerous studies have confirmed the superiority of clomipramine over placebo in these patients, while other antidepressant medications with less potent inhibitory effects on serotonin reuptake (e.g., amitriptyline, imipramine, desipramine) appear to be ineffective. The development of SSRIs fluoxetine, sertraline, paroxetine and fluvoxamine, and their demonstrated anti-OCD actions, support the hypothesis that the anti absorbent effects of these various pharmacological agents are due to their potent

Effects of Serotonin and Dopamine in Obsessive Compulsive Disorder

serotonin reuptake blocking activity.

The hypothesis that SSRIs function in OCD by serotonergic mechanism is also supported by studies that show a strong positive correlation between the improvement of obsessive compulsive symptoms during treatment with clomipramine and the pharmacologically induced decrease in the levels of 5-HIAA 5-hydroxyindolacetic acid serotonin metabolite), and the concentration of serotonin in platelets. Thus, peripheral markers of serotonin function link the improvement of the symptoms of OCD produced by SSRIs to changes in the function of this neurotransmitter (5-HT). However, these markers do not consistently show abnormal serotonergic function in patients with non-treated OCD. Up to 40% of OCD patients no longer respond to SSRIs. In addition, at least some do not demonstrate convincing deregulation of serotonin function. Therefore, other neurotransmitters may be involved in the pathophysiology of OCD in at least some patients with this disorder.

Several lines of evidence demonstrate that dopamine (DA)

is involved in mediating some obsessive compulsive behaviors. Animal studies suggest that high doses of various dopaminergic agents, such as amphetamine, bromocriptine (Parlodel), apomorphine and L-DOPA (Sinemet), induce stereotyped movements in animals, resembling the compulsive behaviors of patients with OCD. Increased dopaminergic transmission may be responsible for this. Studies in humans consistently report that abuse of stimulants such as amphetamine can cause behaviors that appear to be unreasonable, complex and repetitive, similar to the behaviors observed in OCD. Cocaine may also worsen compulsive symptoms in patients with chronic motor disorders of tics such as Tourette's syndrome (TS). The major support for the role of DA in mediating OCD symptoms comes from the relationship of the symptoms of OCD with various neurological disorders associated with DA dysfunction in the basal ganglia (eg, von Economo encephalitis, TS and Sydenham chorea).

Most intriguing is the link between TS and obsessive compulsive symptoms. TS is a chronic neuropsychiatric disorder

Effects of Serotonin and Dopamine in Obsessive Compulsive Disorder

characterized by multiple motor and vocal tics. Between 45% and 90% of TS patients also have obsessions and compulsions. If OCD symptoms were considered separately, a high percentage of patients with TS would be included in OCD diagnostic criteria. Family genetic studies show that TS and OCD are linked, leading to propositions that a common genetic factor may manifest as tics in some individuals and as obsessions and compulsions in others. Put differently, perhaps "tics" are behavioral manifestations of genetic dysfunction located in the basal ganglia, with TS manifesting as "body tics" and OCD as "tics of the mind." Also in support of the involvement of dopamine in the pathophysiology of OCD are the observations that neuroleptic therapy (which blocks DA receptors) added to SSRI treatment reduces the severity of OCD symptoms in patients resistant to SSRI alone, especially in those with concomitant TS.

The serotonergic-dopaminergic hypothesis of OCD: Based on the studies involving serotonin and dopamine in OCD, it seems possible that, at least in some forms of OCD (eg, OCD with TS history), the neurotransmitter systems, both dopamine, and serotonin, may be involved in the pathophysiology of symptoms. Whether the primary abnormality is in serotonin function, in the function of dopamine, or in the balance between the two, is still unclear. This hypothesis is supported by many preclinical data that suggests the existence of important anatomical and functional interactions between the serotonergic and dopaminergic neurons. Thus, it may be that decreases in tonic-inhibitory influences of serotonin on dopaminergic neurons may lead to increased dopaminergic function due to functional connections between dopaminergic and serotonergic neurons in the basal ganglia. Patients with OCD and TS history may thus represent a subtype of the disorder with two neurotransmitters, the balance between them being involved in the pathophysiology of the symptoms.

In summary, the hypothesis that an abnormality in the functioning of neurotransmitters underlies OCD has generated numerous studies on the neuronal systems of serotonin and

Effects of Serotonin and Dopamine in Obsessive Compulsive Disorder

dopamine. To date, consistent neurotransmitter dysfunctions that adequately explain the neurobiological basis of OCD have not been described. However, it seems clear that changes in serotonergic neuronal systems are caused by the known therapeutic agents for OCD, which suggests an important role of serotonin in mediating responses to treatment of this disorder.

<u>Neuroanatomy of OCD:</u> Abnormalities in positron emission tomography (PET scans) images of neuronal activity from cortical projections to the basal ganglia have been confirmed by several researchers in patients with OCD. Specifically, projections from the orbitofrontal cortex may be implicated in OCD. Such abnormalities demonstrated by PET scans in cortical projections to the basal ganglia may even be related to the severity of symptoms; they decrease as patients improve, regardless of whether this improvement occurs after pharmacological treatment or after behavioral therapy.

6 DISCUSSION

Serotonin and obsessive compulsive disorders

Serotonin (5-HT) is a biogenic amine belonging to the group of indoleamines. Chemically, it is constituted by an indole ring, formed by the fusion of a ring benzene and another pyrrolic, and by a side chain ethylamine. It was discovered in extracts of intestinal mucosa and in plasma. Following his discovery in mammalian brain (Amin and Cols, 1954) the possibility was immediately considered that it could act as a neurotransmitter in the central nervous system (CNS). Nowadays it is known that 5-HT meets the requirements of a chemical compound so that it can be considered as a cerebral neurotransmitter. 5-HT is located in specific neurons from which it can be released by an adequate depolarizing stimulus, it produces recordable effects on the neuronal excitability and finally, their actions can be mimicked or blocked by drugs that act on specific recognition sites (Del Rio, 1989).

The use of biochemical fluorescence techniques, as well

as the most recent immunocytological techniques, has allowed the visualization of the different pathways of serotonergic agents existing in the CNS (Emerson, 1983). The cell bodies of the serotoninergic neurons are located exclusively in the brain stem, in groups existing in the bulb (Bl-B4), bulge (B5-B6) and mesencephalon (B7-B9). The biggest part of these being the nuclei of the brainstem raphe since groups BI-B3 are projected nerve fibers to the spinal cord. The cerebellum receives innervation from the groups mesencephalic B7 and B8, and possibly also of the B6 groups of the protuberance. The ascending serotoninergic fibers can be divided into three sections: a) a medial route that starts from the protuberant and mesencephalic raphe (B5-B8) and that innervates mainly the hypothalamus and the preoptic area; b) a lateral route that starts from the mesencephalic raphe (B7-B9) and that fundamentally innervates the cortical areas; and c) a more lateral path that starts from the same mesencephalic nuclei as before and that innervates the extrapyramidal motor system (Azmitia and Segal, 1978).

The receptors for 5-MT were initially classified in the periphery in two subtypes: fundamental, D and M (Gaddmum and Picarelli, 1957). In the CNS, they officially ran two different subtypes of recognition sites for 5-HT: the so-called receptors 5-HT1 and 5-HT2 (Peroutka and Snyder, 1979). Currently, it has been found that the 5-Mil receptor comprises four subtypes, which are called lA, 1B, lC, and 1D (Peroutka, 1988). Of these subtypes, receptors are present in the frontal cortex and in the hippocampus of the human being. Electrophysiological studies suggest that the serotonergic autoreceptors located in the cell bodies of the dorsal raphe should be of type 5-1-a (Gonzalez-Heydrich and Peroutka, 1990). The 5-HTlC receptors have been found in the cerebral cortex and in the choroid plexuses (Hoyer et al, 1986a, b). It has been proven, on the other hand, that the central receptors of 5-HT2 are assimilable to the peripheral receptors that Gaddum and Picarelli called D; these receivers have a high affinity for spiperone, are marked by ketanserin, and are localization mainly postsynaptic.

Finally, there has also been found a place in the CNS with a different recognition for serotonin, to which it has been denominated 5-HT3 that, in certain measures, is assimilable to peripheral M receivers (Kilpatrick, et al, 1987). At first, it was thought that the 5-HT2 receptors were homogeneous, but there is data that suggest that these receptors exist in two affinity states (Peroutka, 1985) and/or that the receptors 5-HTIc possibly belong to the class of 5-HT2 receptors (Hoyer, 1988). The 5-HTlA, 5-HT1C, 5-HTlD and 5-HT2 receptors have been found in the hypothalamus of humans, indicating that one or more of these receptors must be related to the mediation of neuroendocrine responses to central serotonergic agents (Pazos et al, 1988; Coccaro et al, 1990). Serotonin is synthesized from tryptophan, which is captured by the nerve ending; tryptophan penetrates the interior and is degraded enzymatically by tryptophan hydroxylase, giving rise to 5-hydroxytryptophan (5-HTp), which by means of an enzyme, the Ievoaminoacid-decarboxylase, will produce serotonin and then stored in vesicles.

When the nervous impulse arrives, the permeability changes ionic membrane, allowing the entry of a calcium ion that, once inside the synaptic termination, reacts with its specific receptor (calmodulin), starting the release of the neurotransmitter that acts on the specific receptors of serotonin. Part of the released serotonin will be recaptured again by a process of active transportation; it is possible that this reuptake process depends on some specific receptors that have an endogenous ligand. Serotonin that is not recapped is captured by the neighboring cells, and therefore being a neuronal regulation of this release process. On the one hand, the recapped serotonin, which enters freely in the cytoplasm, is degraded by the monoamine oxidase (MAO) so that a balance is established between the serotonin which is free in the cytoplasm and the serotonin stored in the vesicles. In the brain there are 2 types of MAO, the MAO-A and the MAO-B; 5-MT is inactivated preferably by the MAO-A. There is regulation through presynaptic receptors, of which are of two types. In the autoreceptors, that is, the receptors that are sensitive to their own neurotransmitter, it stimulates a decrease in the synthesis and the neurotransmitter itself slows down its release. There are other presynaptic receptors which are sensitive to other neurotransmitters, such as noradrenaline, GABA, and dopamine (Cuenca, 1988).

In terms of physiological functions, many have been classically assigned to this neurotransmitter. The role of 5-HT in the inhibitory system of pain control has been widely studied as regards to the descending paths (Bond, 1986). Sewel and Lee (1980), when investigating the effect of pharmacological manipulation of 5-HT in the antinociceptive activity of morphine and two synthetic analogue enkephalins in mice and rats, verified that the central injection of 5-MT and the peripheral pretreatment with clomipramine (CMI) potentiated the analgesia of both morphine and enkephalins synthetics, while peripheral doses of cyproheptadine caused lesions in the middle raphe dorsal, and pretreatment with reserpine attenuated opiate analgesia.

In the group pre-treated with reserpine, central injection of 5-MT restored antinociceptive activity of morphine, suggesting that 5-MT is possibly one of the related amines with the induction of analgesia of morphine and enkephalins; this is in accordance with jobs in which CMI has been useful for the treatment of pain (Beaumont, 1973). The analgesia caused by acupuncture has shown to be reversible with naloxone (Pome-Rantz and Chiu, 1976), then the endorphins and enkephalins must intervene, therefore CMI can increase the effect of pain treatment with acupuncture. The ascending pathways seem to control a large number of physiological functions such as can be the regulation of body temperature, the regulation of sleep (Candle and Fernández-Camacho, 1987), of hunger (Gardier et al, 1989), sexual activity (González et al, 1989), motor activity and learning (Besson, 1983). The 5-MT suffers environmental influences; Asberg et al (1984a) describe how in the same individual, the concentrations of 5-HIAA in the CSF show seasonal variations which could depict an affective disorders. In adult male monkeys, the total amount 5-MT in the blood can also vary by social and environmental factors (Raleigh et al, 1984).

Dominant males have a higher concentration than those subordinate or that live in groups of only males; the gain or loss of social status is accompanied by the corresponding increase or decrease in the total concentration of 5-MT in blood; temporary isolation also reduced levels. Food also has its influence, especially the intake of foods with many proteins which produce a decrease in the absorption of tryptophan, subsequently having to compete with other amino acids. The absorption of tryptophan increases when the diet has more carbohydrates due to the lack of competition and because carbohydrates induce an increase in insulin secretion, resulting in the release of tryptophan from the muscle to blood.

Methods of study of serotonin function

One of the most important strategies is the measurement of the concentration of 5-MT, its precursors: tryptophan and 5-hydroxytryptophan or its metabolite, 5-

hidoxyindolacetic (5-HIÁÁ) in body fluids. In general, the metabolite gives clear information about the replacement of the active substance (Banki and Molnar, 198 la). Regarding the urinary excretion of 5-HIAA, Bertilsson et al (1982) verify that it is not correlated with its level in the CSF nor does it decrease after CMI administration. CSF reflects central alterations since the treatment with antidepressants that inhibit reuptake of 5-MT reduce the 5-HIAA concentrations of CSF (Siwers et al., 1977; Bertilsson et al, 1980). For years, the lumbar puncture has been the main route for this type of research, both in basal conditions and through strategies such as the technique of the probenecid (Van Praag et al, 1970, 1973). This gives more kinetic information since by blocking the 5-HIAA reabsorption of the CSF, it allows the measurement of the increase after administration.

The LCR studies (Lopez-Ibor et al, 1985) have been able to demonstrate a correlation between the low concentrations of 5-HIAA and suicidal tendencies, according to studies prior from other research groups (Bank and Arato, 1983; Asberg and

Cois, 1984b). CSF studies have several methodological problems, among which are factors such as age, sex, body weight, previous treatments, circadian variations and season, chosen a place to perform the puncture, amount extracted, and different techniques of laboratory (Asberg et al, 1984a). Secondly, studies on secretion, circulation, and reabsorption of the CSF (Bulat, 1984) show that the spinal metabolism is overrepresented which does not exactly reflect the central metabolism. Besides, the information obtained from the LCR is punctual with what sometimes does not provide enough information about the metabolism of neurotransmitters. The third difficulty is the obtaining controls and the fact that the lumbar puncture is not a routine exploration in psychiatry.

An alternative approach is to study peripheral models of serotonergic cells, such as platelets, in which the differences in concentration and activity of the enzymes are related to the metabolism of serotonin (Oreland et al, 1981). A third strategy is the study of biochemical changes induced by psychotropic drugs with serotonergic activity. However, most of these drugs are not sufficiently "clean" and have effects on different neurotransmitter systems. For example, chlorimipramine, a potent 5-HT reuptake blocker, is metabolized to dimethyl-chlorimipramine (DCMI), having a more noradrenergic profile. On the other hand, metabolism depends on age, route of administration, concomitant diseases, other treatments, and idiosyncratic factors (Lopez-Ibor, 1982). From the precursors of the 5MT, only 1% of the tryptophan administered orally reaches the brain, after competing in absorption with other amino acids; 5-hydroxytryptophan is not only incorporated into serotonergic neurons but also to noradrenergic neurons (Moir and Eccleston, 1968). The most recent 5-Hl reuptake inhibitor drugs will produce better information, although will always have to be interpreted by taking into account its interference with multiple systems.

Finally, perhaps most promising approach is the so-called neuroendocrine "probes" serotonergic, consisting of the administration of substances that interfere with the activity of 5-MT by measuring the modification of the peripheral concentration of hormones, whose secretion is controlled by hypothalamic factors influenced by serotonin. For example, the secretion of PRL is blocked by dopamine and controlled by a negative "feedback." Several factors increase the effect dopamixuco (noradrenaline, adrenaline, acetylcholine). 5-MT and other factors (such as melatonin or endogenous peptides) produce an opposite effect. So, different drugs that act in the release of 5-HT, reuptake, receptor activity, and metabolism will produce a modification of the secretion of PRL, depending on the metabolic state of the 5-MT, serving as a measure indirect from it (Laackmann and Cois, 1990). 5-MT is able to regulate the secretion of the hypothalamic-pituitary complex. In response, serotonergic agonists secrete several pituitary hormones: prolactin (PRL), adrenocorticotropic hormone (ACTM), growth hormone (GH), and the renin enzyme (Fuller, 1981, Meltzer, 1982, Leong, 1983, Preziosi, 1983).

The relationship comes from studies that use the administration intraventricular 5-MT and electrical stimulation of serotonergic cells in the area of raphe (Advis et al, 1979;

Krulich et al, 1979). Treatment with p-chlorophenylalanine that prevents the synthesis of 5-HT or the surgical injury of the dorsal raphe nuclei, alters the response to serotonergic agonists (Quattrone et al, 1981). It is important to dwell on the ability of 5-MT to stimulate the secretion of pituitary hormones since it is the basis of the neuroendocrine test used in this thesis; by measuring of PRL, GH, and cortisol through the stimulus provoked by the CMI, we will know indirectly the central serotonergic function.

Prolactin: PRL is a pituitary hormone that is synthesized in the anterior pituitary gland. This composed of about 198 amino acids (AA). In the adult, the woman's levels are slightly superior to those of man, but the ranges of both overlap a lot. In the fertile woman, PRL rates rise during the follicular phase, being maximum during ovulation, to then decrease again during the luteal phase (Báckstrém et al. 1982). With the arrival of menopause, the levels of women and men are equalized (Djursing et al, 1981). The secretion of PRL is pulsatile; corticosteroids, biogenic amines, and endorphins begin regulation (Nira, 1985). A woman's secretion of this is seen affected by sleep, with the maximum peak appearing at 5-8 hours after falling asleep, although it rarely exceeds 30 ng/ml (Frantz, 1987). The levels are maintained more or less constant throughout the year. There is a hypothalamic factor inhibiting PRL – Prolactin Inhibiting Enzyme (PIE); it seems that dopamine is the same PIE or at least a primordial part of its structure (Thorner and Evans, 1984). Of the three CNS dopaminergic pathways, mesolimicocortical, nigrostriatal and tuberoinfundibular, only the latter intervenes in the secretion of PRL. Other inhibitory agents are adrenaline, noradrenaline, acetylcholine, histamine, and neuropeptides: gastrin, neurotensin, vasopressin, and bradykinin.

Various substances with pre- and post-synaptic serotonergic activity have the capacity to increase the plasma levels of PRL. The mechanism by which they stimulate secretion of PRL is still controversial, but it does not seem to be related to dopamine (Kaji et al. 1985). Prolactin is released in response to stress; this response can also be mediated by the opioids (Benker et al, 1990). Other stimulating agents of the PRL are GABA, opioids, histamine, and neuropeptides: VIP, substance P, cholecystokinin, neurotensin, and vasopressin.

1) <u>Cortisol</u>: The secretion of cortisol depends on that of the three inter-communicating regions of the body – the hypothalamus, the pituitary gland, and the adrenal gland. Cortisolemia reaches its lowest point towards midnight and its highest point in the early hours of the morning (12-25 ng/ml). 5-HT stimulates the ACTH-releasing hormone cascade (CRE), ACTM-Cortisol. Acetylcholine, histamine, and neuropeptides also stimulate cortisol: vasopressin, angiotensin, cholecystokinin. It is inhibited by the GABA. Precursors of serotonin synthesis: <u>1-tryptophan</u> - the amino acid of the precursor diet of 5-MT synthesis. High oral doses increase the concentration of 5-MT of human blood platelets and increase the main metabolite of 5-HT, 5-HIAA in plasma, CSF and urine; which is indicative of increased synthesis and replacement of the 5-MT.

Investigations in humans that use doses lower than 90 mg/kg do not show a significant increase in PRL plasma (Fraser et al, 1979; Glass et al, 1980; Westenberg et al, 1982), compared with using doses of 90 to 150 mg/kg (Wiebe et al, 1977, Myypa et al, 1979, Woolf and Lee, 1977). Using an intravenous route (more than 100 mg/kg), there are significant increases in plasma on the basal (Charney et al, 1982, Macindoe and Turkinson, 1973). These results suggest that doses greater than 100 mg/kg are required to increase plasma significantly in healthy subjects and that it may even be necessary to administer intravenously to produce such an effect. It is found that the pretreatment with the antagonist serotoninergic methysergide decreases the increase in PRL caused by 1-tryptophan (Macindoe and Turkinson, 1973), suggesting that this increase is mediated by a serotoninergic mechanism. Antagonists of 5-HT2 receptors: ketanserin and ritanserin do not decrease the response of PRL to tryptophan, suggesting that it is mediated mainly by 5-HTl receptors (Price et al, 1990a).

The response of PRL to tryptophan is flattened in depressed patients (Price et al. 1990a), however, Charney et al (1988) obtain increased plasma responses in OCD patient. On the other hand, modifications of OH induced by 1-tryptophan in a large part of the studies (Glass et al, 1980, Hyyppa et al, 1979, Charney et al, 1982, Koulu, 1982) show a significant increase, but not in all (Westenberg et al, 1982; Macindoe and Turkinson, 1973). Similarly, the increase in GH is inhibited when the serotonergic antagonist cyproheptadine is previously used (Fraser et al, 1979). In the case of GH, the dose-response relationship and the relationship with the route of administration is less clear than with the PRL. Thus, there are significant increases in OH after administration of 2 gr of oral 1-tryptophan (Izlyyppa et al., 1979), but there is not after the infusion of 10 gr intravenous (Macindoe and Turkinson, 1973). The effects of 1-tryptophan on cortisol and plasma ACTH are variable.

2) L-5-hydroxytryptophan: The amino acid 1-tryptophan goes into 5-RTp only by action of tryptophan

hydroxylase present in serotonergic neurons; but the 5-HTp, immediate precursor of 5-MT, can be decarboxylated to serotonin by the enzyme aromatic-L-amino-acid decarboxylase. The intravenous administration of 5-HTp to subjects pretreated with an inhibitor of decarboxylase has produced a significant increase in PRL, more pronounced in women than men (Wirtz-Justice et al, 1876; Puhringer et al., 1976; Lancranjan and cols, 1977). After oral administration (200mgs) PRL increased in some studies (Kato et al, 1974, Yoshimura et al, 1973), but not others (Mandwerger et al, 1975; Beck-Peccoz et al, 1976). Regarding GH, the results of the oral administration of 5HTp are diverse. In a study that included a placebo (Mandwerger et al., 1975), the results found significant differences: regarding intravenous administration in subjects pretreated for 3 days with a decarboxylase inhibitor, infusion of 200 mg of 5-HTp produced a significant increase in GH over baseline and also significant with respect to placebo (Puhringer et al, 1976; Lancranjan et al, 1977), and the administration of the serotonergic receptor antagonist, cyproheptadine after 5-Rip decreased the increase in GH (Nakai et al, 1974). The effects of 5-HTp on cortisol and ACTH are variable. Imura et al (1973) show a significant increase of both after 150 mg orally of 5-Rip. In contrast, Westenberg and Cois (1982) could not demonstrate a significant change in cortisol and Meltzer et al (1983a, 1984) found increases of cortisol after oral administration of 200 mg of 5-HTp.

3) <u>Serotonin-releasing agents</u>: Fenfluramine is an anorectic agent similar in structure to amphetamine, but without stimulating properties. Biochemical data indicate that the serotoninergic agonist properties of fenfluramine derive from its ability to produce a rapid release of 5-MT (Trulson and Jacobs, 1976; Kannengieser et al, 1976; Cleinschmidt and Mc Guffin, 1978). It can also inhibit reuptake of 5-Hl (Garattii et al,

1975), and receptor binding studies suggest that both fenfluramine and its main metabolite, norfenfluramine, may have agonist activity, although weak, of the serotoninergic receptor (Garattini et al, 1979).

Depending on the isomer, its action is more or less specific; thus, d-fenfluramine affects 5-HT levels, metabolism, and synthesis, with little effect on the levels of catecholamines. On the contrary, it is valid for 1-fenfluramine (Invernizzi et al., 1986). There are neuroendocrine studies that show that oral or intravenous administration of fenfluramine increases the plasma levels of PRL in healthy controls (Siater et al. 1976; Quattrone et al, 1983; Siever et al, 1984; Casanueva et al, 1984). The elevation was proportional to the dose administered orally (20 to 100 mg); there were increases significant at the dose of 60, 80 or 100 (Quattróne et al, 1983). Two mg of metergoline, a selective serotonergic receptor antagonist, completely block the increase of PRL produced with 60 mg fenfluramine (Quattrone et al, 1983). Fenfluramine also increases the plasma levels of cortisol and ACTH (Lewis and Sherman, 1984); the increments were proportional to the dose used (between 0.5-1.5 mg/kg) and the response significantly flattened with pretreatment with cyproheptadine, while plasma levels of fenfluramine remained unchanged. Similarly, fenfluramine increases the response of cortisol to insulin-induced hypoglycemia (Balestreri and cols, 1975), but does not significantly alter the OH values (Casanueva et al. 1984).

The Lopez-Ibor Jr. group conducted a study of the different clinical subgroups of depressive disorders, included in the so-called "affective spectrum," (Lopez-Ibor et al, 1988b) ranging from anxiety disorders to major depression with melancholy. They found a negative correlation between the increase of PRL and the greater severity of the disorder. This data seems to show the presence in depression of a flattened response of PRL and 01-1 to the stimulus serotonergic; the fact is that this biochemical alteration seems to be present more in depression, classically considered as more endogenous or more severe.

The group of Lopez-Ibor Jr (1989a) has also presented the results obtained with the test of stimulation with fenfluramine in a sample size of 13 (heroin and other abstinent drugs were included in a therapeutic program with naltrexone). Drug addicts had higher basal plasma cortisol levels than the controls and a minor response of cortisol to the serotonergic fenfluramic stimulus. Serotonergic receptor agonists: m-chlorophenylpiperazine (m-CPP) - is of a substituted piperazine that acts directly as a receptor agonist. Serotoninergic M-chlorophenylpiperazine (m-CPP) is a metabolite of the antidepressant trazodone (Caccia et al, 1982). M-CPP produces PRL plasma elevations up to triple the baseline in healthy controls and is dose-dependent (Mueller et al, 1985a).

Animal studies (Silís et al, 1984) show that m-CPP acts on receptors 5-HT1B, and in one study (Aloi et al, 1984) in Rhesus monkeys, it is indicated that the increase of PRL and GH, but not of cortisol, was flattened previously using the antagonist of the serotoninergic receptor metergoline. There is also an increase in the body temperature and on the scales of humor, including euphoria and anxiety (Mueller and cols, 1985a). M-CPP produces altered neuroendocrine responses in animals when there are changes in cerebral serotonergic receptors, behavioral changes, or both (Invernizi et al, 1981). These findings suggest that these compounds can be used to assess possible changes in postsynaptic receptors during the treatment with psychoactive drugs, as well as abnormalities that may be present in some psychiatric disorders.

4) <u>N-N-dimethylpiperazine</u>: is an indolic hallucinogen with agonist serotonergic properties. It increases PRL, GH, and cortisol; these effects are antagonized by

pretreatment with cyproheptadine (Meltzer et al, 1983b).

Serotonin Reuptake Inhibitors: Clomipramine (CMI): Clomipramine

(CMI) is a tricyclic antidepressant with potent effect in the inhibition of the reuptake of 5-HL. Its pharmacological effect is based on prolonging the stay of 5-HT in the synaptic cleft. Who performs the pharmacological action, unlike the selective agonists, is the 5-MT; for that reason, it will act in a non-selective way in the different receivers. The inhibitors of serotonin reuptake, apparently, can also increase serotonergic transmission by desensitization of terminal serotonergic autoreceptors, by decreasing the ability of these autoreceptors to inhibit 5-MT release (Blier et al., 1990). The CMI, in oral administration, is metabolized between 30-70% in the liver before achieving systemic circulation. The CMI is very lipophilic and has a large volume of distribution, being able to concentrate on tissues and organs related to the lipophilic bases so that the plasma levels are low. The DCMI, metabolite of the CMI, is more polar, has a smaller volume of distribution, and a greater plasma half-life.

It has lower serotonergic activity and has a greater effect on the noradrenergic system. The CMI/DCMI ratio is variable among the different subjects depending on the ability of each one to metabolize CMI. There are interactions between CMI and barbiturates, haloperidol, MAOIs, chronic alcohol, and tobacco use (Peters et al, 1990). The use of the intravenous route, instead of the oral one, determines a change in the quotient between levels of the original drug and those of its active metabolite, with an increase in the drug without alteration of its metabolite. When using the intravenous route, the first step is to avoid the hepatic so it can be a good serotoninergic marker (Trimble, 1990). It has been proven in the rat that chronic treatment with CMI increases progressive discharges in the lateral septal nuclei, which receive mainly serotonergic innervation; in other regions, where the serotonergic innervation is very poor, the treatment does not produce changes which suggest that the action of the CMI should be primarily to the interaction with the serotoninergic system (Contreras et al, 1990).

Intravenous administration of 25 mg causes increases in plasma, per vapor studies performed in healthy volunteers (Sones et al, 1977; Laackman et al, 1984a; Schmauss and Laakman, 1981). The elevations of the PRL, however, did not correlate with the CMI plasma concentrations in 12 healthy subjects (Laackman, 1984a). Studies that use oral or intravenous CMI obtain different results.

Francis and Cois (1976), carried out three pilot studies. In the first, after oral administration of 50 mg of CMI to 6 healthy volunteers, they obtained an increase of the PRL in 3 of them at 2 hours; in a second, in 10 healthy volunteers, the administration of 50 mg of CMI produces an increase of the PRL at 2-4 hours of administration; in the third study, in depressed hospitalized patients without treatment, CMI administration caused a significant increase of the PRL at 3-6 weeks of treatment compared to baseline levels, whereas this increase was not observed in patients treated with amitriptyline. Cole et al (1976) administered doses of 200-250 mg of CMI in an intravenous infusion to 21 patients diagnosed with affective disorder; only 4 of them obtained an increase in the levels of PRL. Iones et al (1977) obtained an increase in plasma 4 hours after oral administration of 50 mg of CMI in 4 healthy volunteers. After antidepressant treatment for 28 days in 34 depressed patients, the increase in PRL did not correlate with plasma CMI levels, DCMI or both, and the increase was greater in women than in men.

With respect to OH, there is great individual variability causing increases defined in only 50% of the individuals who presented an increase in PRL (Laackmann et al, 1984a; Laackmann et al, 1977). There remains an open question and it is the lack of correlation between PRL and the plasma CMI concentration; a possible interpretation could be an individual response to this substance that does not depend on the plasma concentration of the drug (Laackmann et al, 1984a). Studies performed with other 5-HT reuptake inhibitor drugs as citalopram, alaproclate, and zimelidine, have not obtained neuroendocrinological significant effects (Sylvalahti et al, 1979); although these and others like fluoxetine produce changes in the PRL in rodents (Fuller, 1981).

Effects in the response of selective serotonin antagonists and other drugs

<u>Hormone selective serotonin agents</u>: Serotonin antagonists, metergoline, cyproheptadine, and methysergide, significantly block the response of PRL and cortisol to 1-tryptophan, to fenfluramine, and to m-CPP. It seems, as it has been demonstrated in rats and primates, that the non-selective antagonist 5-MT1 acts in the 5-MT l sites, since the selective antagonists ketanserin or ritanserin do not block the effects or produce an increase in the response of PRL to 1-tryptophan (Charig et al, 1986; Idzikowski et al, 1987). The responses of PRL, cortisol and (1-tryptophan, S-HIp or fenfluramine increase with the pretreatment with a series of drugs that are supposed to increase the availability of presynaptic 5-HT,

lithium, and CMI (Siater et al, 1976; Meltzer et al., 1984; cols, 1984; Anderson and Cowen, 1986; Glue et al., 1986). It seems that the primary action of lithium in 5-MT can be presynaptic, with several postsynaptic side effects, which has a net effect of increased serotonergic function (Price et al, 1990b).

The response of PRL or cortisol to the m-CPP agonist does not change or decrease during the treatment chronic with CMI (Zohar et al, 1988). The response of PRL to 1-tryptophan decreased after acute but not chronic diazepam administration (Nutt and Cowen, 1987). The increased response of PRL to 1-tryptophan observed after a single dose of ritanserin disappeared when it was administered for two weeks (Idzikowski et al, 1987).

<u>Other indirect tests of central serotonin function</u>: There have been studies in humans of other physiological and behavioral responses to selective serotonergic agents to assess the functional status of central serotonergic subsystems. Temperature is raised by the serotonergic agonist m-CPP in

humans, monkeys, and rats (Murphy et al, 1989a, Aloi et al, 1984, Wozniak et al, 1989), and the S-MT1/5-MT2 antagonist, metergoline (Mueller et al, 1986), blocks this response. The chronic administration of CMI to humans and rats leads to a decrease (downregulation) of the hyperthermic response to m-CPP (Zohar et al, 1988; Wozniak et al. 1989). However, highly selective agonists from other serotonergic sites, especially 8-hydroxy-2 (di-n-propylamino) tetralin (8-OM-DPAT), that acts in place of 5-HT1A in rodents, produces hypothermic effects instead of hyperthermic which are blocked by different antagonists (Gudelsky et al, 1986).

Functional heterogeneity of subsystems in cerebral serotonergic pathways: Higher evidence of this heterogeneity comes from the observation of the hyposensitivity of the temperature and the behavioral response to the Mpmeba effect (Erasto Batholomeo Mpemba, b.1950) with m-CPP after treatment with chronic with CMI; whereas the increased neuroendocrine response (PRL and cortisol plasma) did not vary in magnitude from chronic treatment with CMI (Zohar et al. 1988). Modifications of sleep to selective agents have also been studied for serotonergic, including 1-tryptophan, fenfluramine, trazodone, fluoxetine, zimelidine, indalpine, ritanserin, and m-CPP. The difficulty of sleep found in healthy volunteers with m-CPP (Lawlor et al, 1989) was also observed in rodents, which showed suppression of rapid eye movements (REM) (Pastel and Fernstrom, 1987), in contrast to the slow-wave sleep increased by the 5-HT2 antagonist, ritanserin, again indicating the heterogeneity of serotonergic subsystems in man.

The effects of behavior, cognitive, locomotor, cardiovascular and other selective serotonergic agents are also interesting measures. Again, the anxiogenic effects of some agents such as m-CPP (Charney et al, 1987; Mueller et al, 1986; Mueller et al, 1985b) with the anxiolytic action of drugs that act selectively in other serotonergic receptors such as 5HT1A agonists, buspirone, gepirone, ipsapirone (Traber and Glaser, 1987), and some of the 5-HT2 antagonists such as ritanserin (Ceulemans et al, 1985). One has observed a decrease in the angiogenic response of m-CPP to the chronic administration of CMI (Zohar et al, 1988), as well as the observation of diminished behavioral responses with the age of m-CPP (Lawlor et al, 1989). Serotonin syndrome of behavior has been widely studied in rodents (Jacobs, 1976), has an equivalent effect on humans who receive CMI, while residual effects of treatment with IMAGES persist (Insel and cols, 1982a); a similar phenomenon has been described when tryptophan is administered with MAOIs (Pare, 1963, Thomas and Rubin, 1984).

Usefulness of serotonin agents that interact with different subtypes of receptors in the treatment of neuropsychiatric disorders:

5-HT1a: For many years, it has been speculated that 5-MT is related to the physiology of anxiety. Supporting this point of view are the observations that benzodiazepines decrease the serotonergic neurotransmission (Trulson et al, 1982) and the finding that agonists selective and partial 5-HT1a receptors have anxiolytic effects (Sprouse and Aghajanian, 1988). Clinically, the best results came from a study of buspirone, although also gepirone, ipsapirone, and SM-3997 have been studied in clinical trials (Feighner and Boyer, 1989). Buspirone is a partial agonist of the 5-HT1a receptors, for which it has a high affinity and some selectivity (Peroutka, 1985). Some properties of 5-HT1a receptors and their agonists in animals suggest that it can be effective antidepressants; chronic antidepressant treatment produces a reduction of 5-HT1a receptors in rodents and also of 5-Mi receptors. (Gonzalez-Heydrich and Peroutka, 1990). Chronic treatment with buspirone or gepirone produces a similar reduction of 5-HT2 receptors. Recent clinical trials (Robinson et al, 1989) in patients with depression find buspirone and gepirone more effective than placebo in reducing depression per Hamilton's score of anxiety.

5-HT1a agonists may also be useful in the treatment of alcoholism. It has been verified that the activation of 5-MT decreases the consumption of alcohol and the deficit of recent memory loss (Tollefson, 1989). At least in one study, (Bruno, 1989) the treatment with buspirone in alcoholic patients was better than placebo in terms of the continuation of treatment, decreased appetite for alcohol, and overall psychopathological improvement. Other potential uses of 5-HT1a agonists include appetite regulation, intake of food, and the treatment of hypertension (Gilbert and Dourish, 1987).

<u>5-HT1D</u>: 5-HT1D receptors are extended in the human brain, in or near the cerebral blood vessels. An agonist of 5-HT1D receptors, sumatriptan, has been seen to produce vasoconstriction of the cerebral arteries (Feniuk et al, 1987). Recently, it has been described as being extremely effective in the acute treatment of a migraine and that it causes minimal side effects.

5-HT2: The role of 5-HT2 receptors in depression is not clear. The classical antidepressant drugs decrease the number of 5-HT2 receptors in the cerebral cortex of the rat (Peroutka and Snyder, 1980). Two receptor antagonists are being studied, mianserin and nefazodone, in the USA, for use as antidepressants (GonzalezHeydrich and Peroutka, 1990). Both chronic and acute treatment with mianserin decreases the density of 5-HT2 receptors, especially in the frontal cortex. The 5-HT2 antagonists may also be useful in the treatment of anxiety disorders as suggested by its effectiveness in a number of animal anxiety measures (Chopin and Briley, 1987). The efficacy of mianserin in the treatment of anxiety has been described as "generalized," but not in panic disorders (Westenberg and den Boer, 1989). The most studied of the antagonists is its prophylactic efficacy for migraines. It has been proven as effective in patients as with methysergide, pizotifen, cyproheptadine, and lisuride.

The effect of 5-HT2 antagonists, such as cyproheptadine, has also been studied with results leading to an increase in appetite and weight gain in patients with anorexia nervosa (GonzalezHeydrich and Peroutka, 1990). Ritanserin, a serotonin receptor antagonist which was never marketed for clinical use but has been used in scientific research, has been shown to increase significantly the slow waves of sleep (Idzikowski et al, 1987). Other 5-HT2 antagonists such as ketanserin have also been studied in some cardiovascular diseases and peripheral vascular diseases, thrombotic and embolic episodes, and cardiopulmonary emergencies.

5-HT3: Antagonists of this receptor, such as ICS 205-930, MDL 72222, BRL 24924 and ondansetron, have powerful antiemetic effects in animals and in man (Fozard, 1987), improving nausea and vomiting induced by chemotherapy. Another possible indication of antagonist 5-HT3 is the treatment of gastrointestinal disorders of motility caused by the overproduction of 5-MT. Possible utilities of psychotherapeutic agents of 5-MT3 antagonists include their usefulness as antinoise agents and antipsychotics. Its possible use in psychosis is suggested by the inhibitory effect of 5-HT3 antagonists in the dopaminergic function (Kilpatrick et al, 1987).

<u>Serotonin reuptake inhibitors</u>: These drugs (fluvoxamine, fluoxetine, paroxetine, citalopram, indalpine, zimelidine and sertraline) have been shown to be effective in improvement of depression, panic attacks, and OCD. Also, they seem to be effective in the treatment of obesity, substance abuse, and sleep disorders (Gonzalez-Heydrich).

Disease	Possible 5-MT receiver (s) related
Anxiety	5-HT1A, 5-HT2, 5-HT3
Depression	5-HTlA, 5-H922, 1 • recap. 5-HT
OCD	1 recapture 5-HT
Migraine (acute)	5-HT1D
Migraine (prophylaxis)	5-HT2
Suppression of appetite	5-HTlA, intake system.

Table 1: Summary of clinical indications of drugs that act on the Serotonin Receptors.

Serotonin and Psychopathology

Since the introduction of antidepressants into psychiatric practice, specialists have observed that not all symptoms respond in the same way to different drugs. Eastern medicine adopted the concept formulated by Freyhan in 1960 (Freyhan, 1979) of target symptoms, which can be defined as the result of the observation that not all psychopathological facts and symptoms presented in a patient respond in the same way or with the same rapidity to the application of the psychopharmaceutical. The first investigations in this line are those of Banki et al (1977, t981a, 1981b, 1981c, 1981d, 1983, 1984) who, in a mixed group of psychiatric patients (major depression, schizophrenia, adjustment disorders and alcoholism), found relationships between certain clinical features and the low concentration of certain neurotransmitter metabolites in the CSF, regardless of the category diagnostic. The most significant correlations were those between suicide attempts and 5-HIAA; and delirious symptoms, psychomotor inhibition, and homovanillic acid (a metabolite of dopamine).

It is in suicide that a more direct relationship with serotonin has been demonstrated; the postmortem studies show an increase in the number of 5-HT2 receptors, postsynaptic, in the frontal cortex of suicidal victims (Stanley and Mann, 1983); Arora and Meltzer (1989) detected a greater number of 5-HT2 receptors in 32 suicides than in 37 controls deceased by other causes. Furthermore, the increase in 5-HT2 receptors was significantly higher in violent suicides than in non-violent suicides. In victims of suicide, Korpi et al (1986) find a low concentration of 5-HT in the hypothalamus. A decrease in the binding sites of imipramine has been observed in serotoninergic endings of the frontal cortex of suicidal victims (Stanley and Gershon, 1982; Perry et al, 1983), there was a decrease in the activity of MAO in alcoholics who committed suicide (Gottfries et al, 1975), and a decrease was found in the blood platelets of suicidal patients (Meltzer and Arora, 1990). Chronic treatment with certain antidepressants causes a reduction in the density of 5-HT2 receptors (Peroutka and Snyder, 1980). All these findings suggest a decreased, presynaptic, serotonergic activity leading to compensatory regulation and increased postsynaptic binding sites (Stanley and Stanley, 1990). The antidepressant treatment could act by reducing the number of 5-Mi receptors, which would allow for a normalization of the balance between presynaptic and postsynaptic receptors, and recovery of central serotonergic function. However, not all postmortem studies are concordant, thus Gross-Isseeroff et al (1989) found no significant differences between controls and suicide victims regarding the binding sites of imipramine in the cortex prefrontal, whereas Meyerson et al (1982), on the contrary, found them increased.

It is considered that a low level of 5-HIAA in the CSF is a possible predictor of subsequent suicides (Asberg et al, 1986) and more frequent hospitalizations in the case of affective disorders (van Praag and De Haur, 1979). Sones and Cois (1990) observed that in elderly patients who made suicide attempts, the 5-HIAA levels of CSF were significantly lower than in a control group of elderly people with no history of attempts suicidal; however, they did not detect differences with respect to measures that they valued psychosocial, psychological or behavioral factors, which supports the idea that psychological factors are less useful when assessing suicidal risk in the elderly. Some authors suggest that the relationship between suicidal behavior and 5-HIAA has to be with aggressive behavior in general. In animals, an inverse relationship has been described between central serotonergic function and aggression (Kulkarrú, 1968; Sewel et al, 1982). Kent et al (1988) found a strong inverse relationship between impulsivity and decrease in uptake of 5-HT by platelets, which represents the presynaptic serotonergic function of the CSF. The relationship between 5-HIÁA and suicidal behavior has also been seen in affective disorders (Brown et al, 1982; Brown and Goodwin, 1984); in patients schizophrenics who were not depressed (Van Praag, 1983; Levy et al., 1984; Ninan and cols, 1984) and personality disorders (Brown et al, 1982). Greenberg and Coleman (1976) found the 5-HIAA decrease in CSF associated with hyperactivity and aggressive behavior in children. Kmesi et al (1990) found diminished levels of 5-HIAA in the LCR of children and adolescents with behavioral disorders.

Regarding aggressiveness, they use as a control group

patients with OCD, where the levels found are higher. Linnoila et al (1983) observed that criminals who were violent and impulsive, compared to those who had meditated and prepared the violent criminal action, had lower concentrations of 5-HIAA in the LCR. Equally decreased levels of 5-HIAA were found in patients who made attempts to suicide after killing their children (Lidberg et al, 1984). Traskman and Cols (1981) found that the 5-HIAA levels of CSF were significantly lower only between those who had committed an attempted violent suicide (hanging, sticking a shot, throwing out the window, gas, deep cuts) compared to attempts not violent (drug intoxication). Bioulac et al (1980) found this decrease in criminals with syndrome 47, XYY, institutionalized for violence and aggression, and where the substitution treatment with 5-HTp normalized the metabolism of serotonin and attenuated enormously clinical symptomatology. Virkkunen and Cols (1987) found it in arsonists that meet DSM-III criteria for borderline personality disorder. The finding is interesting of the correlation between low concentrations of 5-HIAA in the

CSF and the hostility scores of the Rorschach (Rydin et al, 1982), or with impulsivity and behavior "seeker of sensations" (Oreland et al, 1981). Roy and Linnoila (1988) have verified the existence of a negative correlation between the levels of 5-HIAA and the score obtained on the acting-out subscale, contained in a question of hostility in healthy volunteers. Coccaro et al (1986) found flat responses to fenfluramine in personality disorders with physical aggression and motor impulsivity.

A doctoral thesis on serotonergic mechanisms in the control of impulses using a 5-MT agonist, di-fenfluramine, in non-depressive multi-impulsive patients, gets flattened responses from both PRL and cortisol. Cocaro et al (1989) described a strong relationship between the history of aggressive/impulsive behavior, suicide attempts, consumption of alcohol and response of the PRL to fenfluramine, which may indicate a decrease of the serotonergic response of the hypothalamic-pituitary-adrenal axis in human aggression (Brown and Linnoila, 1990). Each author has shown that the concentration of 5-HIAA in CSF and the response of TSH to TRiH presents a significant inverse correlation (Arato et al, 1983; Banki et al. 1984; Lopez-Ibor, Jr et al, 1985). Serotonin is involved in the regulation of secretion of TSH (Collu, 1979) by inhibiting its secretion; a central serotoninergic hypoactivity could be reflected in the low concentration of 5-HIAA in the CSF and at the same time in the increased TSH response to TRH, and consequently both could be related to the facilitation of aggressive behavior or violent suicide. Roy et al (1986a) found that the combination of 5-HIAA decreased in the CSF and the response of the suppression test of the abnormal dexamethasone predicts suicide better than such measurements separately.

Norman et al (1990) corroborate in their study for the usefulness of DST for monitoring of the risk of suicide after hospital discharge. Virkkunen (1982, 1983, 1984) showed that the violent individuals had hyperinsulinemia and went on to hypoglycemia after oral glucose overload; these anomalies were more evident in those subjects with traits of more severe and chronic personality disorder, and also presented insomnia problems, suggesting an alteration of the circadian cycle. In rats, the lesion of the nuclei suprachiasmatic, which receives a serotonergic entry from the nuclei of the raphe, causes hyperinsulinemia, hypoglycemia and alterations of the circadian rhythm (Yamamoto and cols, 1985). Yaryura-Tobias and Neziroglu (1978) studied a group of 12 patients who presented aggressive behavior, obsessive compulsive symptoms, and self-mutilations, along with insomnia and severe sexual disorders, 9 of which had a past history of anorexia nervosa and all of them had impaired glucose tolerance curves; these authors note that a large part of the symptoms and signs of their patients have been identified in the pathophysiology of the hypothalamus (diabetes mellitus, sleep disturbances and of appetite, violent behavior and amenorrhea due to stress) which contains relatively high concentrations of 5 MT, and all these patients improved by being treated with CMI.

Greater evidence of the serotoninergic component in

impulsivity and aggression comes from pharmacological studies. Depletion of 5-MT by injury or drugs can provoke aggressive or impulsive behaviors (uninhibited) in animals (Soubrie, 1986); the potentiation of serotonergic activity following the administration of tryptophan, 5-HTP, MAOIs and serotonergic receptor stimulators, reduce or abolish aggression in isolated mice (Modge and Butcher, 1974). The administration of tryptophan and serotonin also suppresses the aggression produced by intrahypothalamic microinjections of acetylcholine (Állikmets, 1974). In humans, drugs such as ethanol and benzodiazepines can also cause disinhibition, impulsivity, and aggressiveness; ethanol has complex effects that depend on the time of the turn-over of the 5-MT and the acute (non-chronic) administration of benzodiazepines may reduce serotonergic function (Nutt et al, 1986). The administration of 5-HTP, the precursor of 5-MT, appears to be effective in controlling self-mutilation in Lesch-Nyhan syndrome (Mizuno and Yasumi, 1974).

These works and others present in the literature

provide more and more conclusive data to relate human suicide and interpersonal aggression to the central metabolism of serotonin (López-Ibor et al, 1989b). On the other hand, considering the systems of serotonergic and noradrenergic neurotransmission as interacting provides us with a more accurate information on biochemistry, CNS impairment, behavior, and experience with auto aggressiveness, than if we think of serotonin as an isolated component. A biochemical imbalance could create a vulnerability that could become the basis of the aggressive-type phenomenon. The drugs that enhance 5-HT, in particular, 5-HTP, increase the synthesis of 5-MT and 5-HT reuptake inhibitors, such as CMI, trazodone, fluvoxamine, and fluoxetine; they have also been shown to have therapeutic effects in panic disorders (Koczkas et al, 1981; Kahn et al, 1987; Khan and Westenberg, 1985; Evans et al. 1986; Den Boer et al, 1987; Ayuso and Ayuso, 1989). There is no data available on the 5HIAA in the CSF in patients with panic disorder; but in depressed patients, it has observed a negative relationship between 5-HIAA in the CSF and anxiety levels (Van Praag, 1988).

These publications suggest the importance of serotonergic transmission in apparently very different behaviors such as suicide, aggression, and lack of impulse control. This hypothesis can explain the findings in bulimics, alcoholism, or in behaviors where the lack of control of impulses seems evident. In the case of pathological players, a response has been obtained whereas PRL flattens to the stimulus of the CMI (Moreno, 1991). In bulimia, Brewerton et al (1986) have found a flattening of the PRL to m-CPP, and Kaye and Cols (1984) have observed lower levels of 5HIAA in anorexics with bulimia than in anorexics without bulimia. In patients with a dependence on alcohol, who have been abstaining for a few weeks, low CSF 5-HIAA levels were found (Ballenger et al 1979; Borg et al, 1985; Banki, 1981d); these patients as a group are known to have a high risk of suicide (Roy and Linnoila, 1986b) and many of them are impulsive, especially under the influence of alcohol (Linnoila et al, 1983). Branchey et al (1984) show that the relationship between tryptophan and neutral amino acids in the blood is lower in alcoholics with a prior history of aggressive/impulsive and/or suicidal behavior.

These authors find a relationship statistically significant between aggressive and suicidal behavior in the same individuals. The relationship between tryptophan and neutral amino acids is important because it is thought to regulate the amount of tryptophan, the amino acid of the 5-Rl precursor diet, which is transported through the blood-brain barrier to the brain for the synthesis of 5-HT (Brown and Linnoila, 1990). In a study by Jensen and Garfinkel (1988) on evolutionary data of 31 adults who during their childhood had been consulted for hyperactivity, distractibility and/or impulsivity, they were reevaluated at 21-23 years and a negative correlation was found between the activity of the MAO enzyme in platelets and the consumption of alcohol, the provocation of fires and the "Search for sensations" according to the scale of Zuckerman. The findings in OCD could fit with this hypothesis since in obsessions, the impulse control problem is important and becomes evident when the rituals of the patient are not effective enough, and violent behavior occurs auto or heteroagresiva (Lopez-Ibor, 1988c). Coursey, in a 1984 review about the dynamic aspects of OCD, studied the different scales of the Rorschach test completed by patients suffering from this pathology, observing that the hostile impulses and sadists are the main component of this disorder. There are few published studies on the levels of 5-HIÁÁ in the CSF of patients with OCD. In one study, you find an increase in levels (Insel et al., 1985), and in another, there is a tendency to increase in CSF 5-HIAA levels (Thoren et al, 1980b).

These results, if not well corroborated in larger samples, could have phenomenological implications. A characteristic feature of patients with OCD is the pathological guilt, that is, a fault in absence of fault. In this aspect, the obsessive compulsive individual is exactly opposite to the sociopath, who performs aggressive, criminal acts of impulsive and lacks feelings of guilt. In the studies that we have reviewed previously in aggressive and impulsive patients, we found 5-HIAA levels in the LCR decreased, contrary to that observed in patients with OCD, which can be characterized by a strict control of their aggressive impulses. The fact that, in spite of the suffering patients have with OCD, a very small number of patients commit suicide. Of special interest in the phenomenology of OCD, is the evidence (Trioso and Sehino, 1986) that the increase of substitute behaviors in social groups of rodents and primates which may be associated with the subordinate or the expired. The subordinate members of primate social groups are characterized by a single behavioral, endocrine and neurochemical event, which is the increase of 5-HIAA in the LCR when compared with non-subordinate members of the group (Winslow and Insel, 1990).

In other disorders, it has been seen (for example) that patients with Parkinson's syndrome show low levels of 5-HIAA in the CSF had a higher incidence of depression and suicidal behavior (Brown and Linnoila, 1990). Individuals with alterations in the metabolism of steroids, for example with Cushing's syndrome, affect the metabolism of 5-MT and have a higher incidence of depression and suicidal behavior (Lewis and Smith, 1983). In the syndrome Gilles de la Tourette, which is also characterized by aggressive behavior, it has been described to have an association with low levels of 5-HIAA in the CSF (Cohen et al, 1978). Also, they have found alterations of 5-MT in Attention Deficit Disorders (Irwing and Cois, 1981), "minimal brain dysfunction" (Wender, 1969) and psychotic syndromes in childhood (Campbell et al, 1974), and in other CNS-related disorders such as phenylketonuria (Pare and cols, 1957), Alzheimer's disease, and epilepsy. O'Neil et al (1986) describe the presence of low levels of 5-MT in blood in a 22-year-old man, mentally retarded with Cornelia de Lange syndrome, that presented alterations in sleep, auto behavior and hetero-aggressive, and how treatment with tryptophan and trazodone improved sleep and conduct. In migraines and asthma, a decrease in 5-MT uptake has been found in platelets (Malmgren et al, 1980); Traskman-Bendz (1988) found that psychiatric patients with low levels of 5-HIAA in the CSF had first-degree relatives who had asthma in a greater proportion than those patients with high levels of 5-HIAA.

Neuroimaging techniques in obsessive compulsive disorders

The appearance of functional imaging techniques has represented an important advance in the ability to understand the normal and abnormal functioning of the brain. Currently, Positron Emission Tomography (PET) remains the technique that provides the most information, since it allows to quantify the blood flow and metabolism in the brain, in addition to having a higher quality spatial resolution. The introduction of PET several decades ago has allowed us to show a lot of functional alterations in psychiatric and neurological diseases, including cerebrovascular pathology, cerebral degenerative diseases, and epilepsy. Perhaps the next big challenge for PET could be finding neurobiological determinants for various non-organic mental disorders since in general there is no doubt that psychiatric diseases are fundamentally due to alterations in the normal functioning of the brain. Cerebral perfusion

SPECT offers a wide potential for the investigation of the etiopathogenesis and physiopathology of psychiatric disorders. On the other hand, and more recently with the cerebral SPECT of neuroreceptors, it is possible to study the density, distribution, and degree of occupation of CNS receptors and neurotransmission systems involved in psychiatric diseases.

The cerebral SPECT in psychiatry continues being only a technique primarily for research, although work is being done to define its practical clinical usefulness. The lack of specificity of regional brain dysfunctions measured by SPECT for a psychiatric pathology determines that current applications in psychiatry are limited to the evaluation of patients with an atypical clinical finding and the differential diagnosis of certain psychiatric syndromes. In any case, SPECT results should always be interpreted together with the data and these should, in turn, be integrated with the current knowledge of the pathophysiology of each entity. Only in this way will it be possible to determine the meaning of the functional information provided by SPECT in the field of psychiatry.

Studies with computerized axial tomography in obsessive compulsive disorders: Luxemberg et al. (1988) analyzed the brain volume of ten patients who suffered OCD, all males, and ten controls matched by age; they found that the volume of the caudate nucleus was significantly lower in the patients, but there was no difference in other hemispheric structures or in the ventricles. However, Insel et al (1983), in a sample of ten patients and controls found no significant differences.

Stein and colleagues, in 1993, designed a study comparing patients with OCD with a high score on the scale of Minor Neurological Signs (MNS) to patients with OCD and a low score on that scale. Both groups were compared with a control group matched in age and sex. All patients underwent a CAT scan. The different neuroanatomical structures were measured using a quantitative volumetric analysis. Patients with a high score on the MNS scale had an increase statistically significant in the volume of the ventricles compared to patients with a low score and in the control group. The caudate and ventricular nuclei did not present differences between these groups.

Magnetic resonance studies in obsessive compulsive disorders: Weilburg et al. (1989) report a single patient with obsessive compulsive symptomatology, in which the MRI showed a marked decrease in the volume of the head of the left caudate, with an increase in size in the left lateral ventricle and abnormalities in the lateral putamen. However, this patient had an atypical clinical finding since she suffered auditory and olfactory pseudohallucinations, as well as postures dystonic and asymmetric hypertonia, with what could be a case of OCD being a secondary diagnosis, since she also had a history of brain dysfunction from childhood. Garber et al. (1989) studied a group of thirty-two subjects with OCD and a control group. The right frontal white matter had alterations in the Ti relaxation time. Those who had a positive family history of OCD presented more negative differences in the right-left Ti values in the anterior cingulate gyrus. In addition, there was a significant correlation of right-left differences for Ti in the orbital cortex. These differences varied according to the

Effects of Serotonin and Dopamine in Obsessive Compulsive Disorder symptomatology, according to if the patients took medication or not, and if they had a family history of OCD. The time is proportional to the mobility of water protons in membranes and fluids and may reflect an increase in free water or decrease in the molecular binding of water, which can be secondary to alterations of the extracellular or cytoplasmic membrane, or even to alterations in blood flow or CSF. The authors suggest a possible involvement of the serotoninergic projections of the frontal cortex via the cingulate or the stretched.

In the study of the Laplane group (1989) on obsessive disorder resulting from injuries in the basal ganglia (for several causes such as poisoning by monoxide carbon, alcohol, or even after the sting of a wasp), seven of the eight patients presented lesions in general in the lentiform nucleus, particularly affecting the pale, and with generalized cerebral atrophy in two cases. However, particular characteristics of this group do not make it comparable with other studies. Charles et al. (1990) studied a group of twelve patients with obsessive compulsive disorder and a group of twelve controls matched in age and sex. Everyone had an MRI and they found no statistically significant differences in the head of the caudate nucleus, cingulate, corpus callosum. This data is limited and cannot rule out the presence or absence of a structural normality in OCD patient. However, Scarone et al. in 1991, found an increase in the size of the right nucleus caudate in patients with OCD with respect to a control group. The sample was formed by twenty patients and a matched control group in age and sex of twelve patients. The findings showed no correlation with demographic, psychopathological or clinical data.

Calabrese et al. (1992) found a statistically significant increase in the size of the right caudate nucleus using a sample of twenty patients who met criteria for DSM-III-r for OCD (eight males, twelve females) and a control group of fourteen subjects (eight males and six females). The intensity of the MRI signal was measured in time; relaxation Tí showing statistically significant differences between the left and right caudate nucleus, the left being greater. This asymmetry did not appear in the group control. Ienike et al. (1992) answered this publication by proposing a study with several imaging techniques (PET, NMR, and spectroscopy by NMR) to evaluate the neurosurgical treatment of OCD patients resistant to other treatments.

Studies with PET scans in obsessive compulsive disorder patients

In Positron Emission Tomography (PET) scans, the subject is injected with a radiopharmaceutical marked with a radionuclide that emits positrons (in the case of the brain, it is fluorodeoxyglucose), that when it reaches the tissue, it will emit electrons of matter constituent of the subject, which will then release two gamma rays for each positron in the opposite direction (~180 degrees) that, when they can be detected, allow quantification and exact location of the injected substance and the preparation of tomographies of a high resolution. In 1987, Baxter, Lewis, and Cois published the first work with PET scans in patients with OCD compared the metabolic rates of 14 patients using the Fi8-FDO as a marker (fluoro-deoxyglucose), with 14 depressed patients of unipolar type without OCD, and with 14 healthy controls. They found that patients with OCD had metabolic rates significantly higher in the left gyrus orbitalis, as well as in both caudate nucleus, and there were also alterations in the right "girus orbitalis" with a tendency not statistically significant. Of the fourteen patients, ten were evaluated after treatment with trazodone; these patients showed a decrease in glucose metabolism rates, although these were also not statistically significant.

The ratio between glucose consumption between the caudate and the rest of the ipsilateral hemisphere significantly increased in patients who responded to treatment. This study presents a problem in the methodology - since five patients were being treated with neuroleptics, tranquilizers, or antidepressants, and this was not taken into account, the co-morbidity is that some of the cases had a depression associated to OCD. In addition, as Pigtt et al (1992) point out, trazodone has a weak anti-obsessive action, which may explain that in combination with other drugs, the anti-obsessive effect may find statistically significant differences. One year later, this same group compared a sample of ten patients with OCD which were untreated at least two weeks before the PET scan to ten healthy controls. They find a greater metabolism of glucose in the flows, in the gyrus orbitalis, and in the ratio of this to the ipsilateral hemisphere when taken together. Therefore, the findings of this study are bilateral. Another observation in this study is that men have superior glucose consumption rates on the left side and women on the right.

In 1989, Nordahl et al. studied sixty areas of interest in eight patients during the performance of an auditory task, finding higher rates of metabolism in both orbital areas. In animal and human studies, it showed that repeated administration of painful electrical currents increased the consumption of glucose in the orbital region. These authors think that the orbital cortex may be involved in habituation, extinction, and in inhibition and that a pathological dysfunction at that level can lead to a clinical appearance similar to OCD.

Swedo et al. (1989) examined eighteen patients with PET scan, nine of each sex, who present OCD since childhood, finding an increase in metabolism in the left orbitofrontal region, left motor-sensory cortex, in the anterior bilateral "girus cínguli," and in the bilateral prefrontal areas. However, the activity in the right orbital cortex correlates with the severity of the disorder and possibly with the response to treatment.

In a study published in 1990, Martinot et al. found a reduced consumption of glucose in the frontal regions including medial and lateral prefrontal orbital, as well as in the striate and thalamus. Benkelfart et al. (1990) found that after a response to treatment with CMI, PET scans indicate that the decrease in glucose consumption that best relates to the response was the left caudate, with minor variations on the right side. The group of Thoren, in 1988, showed that the effect of the CMI on acid concentrations in CSF depended on the degree of serotonergic inhibition exerted: below of 50%, the level of HVA in CSF is increased, and above is decreased. The CMI acts directly on dopaminergic transmission, in addition to blocking it in the reuptake of serotonin, and has shown that important effects on the indices of glucose consumption of the caudate. In this study, they also found a decrease statistically significant in the consumption of glucose in the orbital cortex when they responded to the treatment.

The group of Sawele and Frackoviack (1991) studied a sample of six patients with OCD using oxygen-lS, and with 18-fluorodopa (to visualize and estimate function dopaminergic). They found an orbitofrontal hypermetabolism in the medial regions, frontal and premotor. They also observed a normal uptake of dopamine in caudate, putamen and frontal medial cortex. In this investigation, the patients presented with an extreme slowness in the execution of routine tasks due to rituals that consumed time, compulsions, or checking behaviors. Lewis, Baxter et al. (1992) analyzed the changes in glucose consumption in different brain areas in relation to the response or resistance to pharmacological treatments with fluoxetine from an initial dose of 20 mg/day increasing to 60-80 mg/day at two weeks, on behavior. When patients respond to any of the treatments, there is a very significant decrease in metabolic activity in the head of the right caudate, but no change when they do not respond to treatment.

The activity of the orbital cortex (before treatment) correlates significantly with that of the caudate and thalamus; this correlation disappears after the therapeutic response. Based on these data, this group raises a theory about the pathophysiology of the disease, suggesting that there would be a brain circuit formed by these structures whose hyperactivity seems to cause the presentation of symptoms. An important consequence of this study is the non-appearance of significant changes in the orbitofrontal regions, contracted to what happens in the study by Swedo et al. (1992), which analyzed changes in PET scans after exclusive treatment with SSRIs. The authors explain it's according to the different duration of the treatments: Baxter et al. says it is ten weeks, while that of Swedo et al. analyzed it is done after one year of treatment, and Benckelfart uses CMI and studies them at sixteen weeks. Thus, differences in metabolic activity in the caudate could precede the cortical. With the treatment, the caudate could be made more efficient in the control of obsessive symptoms and their metabolic changes are not observed, as occurred in the work of Swedo.

Azari et al. (1993) compared a sample of ten patients with OCD before and after a pharmacological treatment with a control group; the cerebral metabolic rate was measured with PET scan. The results showed differences between eight of the ten patients before the treatment while after the treatment 70% of the patients presented images identical to those of the control group. These differences involved the base ganglia, thalamus, the limbic system and cortical association regions. Scott et al. (1994) designed a study to determine neuroanatomical alterations of OCD on a sample of eight patients. These patients underwent a PET scan at rest and another after a stimulation that caused an increase in their symptoms. The stimuli that caused an increase in symptomatology was individualized. The images showed a statistically significant increase in brain blood flow during the symptomatic state in the right caudate nucleus with p <0.006, in left anterior cingulate with p <0.45, and bilaterally in the orbitofrontal cortex with a p <0.08. There was also an increase in flow in the left thalamus, but this was not statistically significant, p=0.07. These findings coincide with previous results in neuroimaging studies in OCD patients.

In summary, PET scan studies for obsessive compulsive disorder show a remarkable coincidence in the results, being the findings compatible with the existence of a dysfunction in the circuits that connect the orbital cortex with the basal ganglia. All these observations are supported by the response to the medical and surgical treatment of the disorder and in the anatomical distribution of serotonergic pathways and cortico-subcortical connections.

Studies with SPECT in obsessive compulsive disorder

Recent advances in psychopharmacology and neuroimaging techniques support the hypotheses on the biological bases of OCD. The anatomical substrate would be involved in the frontal lobe (orbitofrontal cortex), the basal ganglia (caudate nucleus), and the cingulate, which is the region of the frontal lobe that connects with the basal ganglia. SPECT is a functional test that tomographically measures cerebral blood flow by injecting a widely used, marked contrast, HMPAO (hexamethylpropyleneamine oxime), labeled with Technetium 99 metastable, a lipophilic molecule that crosses the blood-brain barrier and is converted to its hydrophilic form after being trapped in the nervous tissue. The HMPAO has the property to provide representative images of the regional cerebral perfusion existing at the time of injection without altering its distribution (at least during the first three hours).

Machlin, Hoehn-Saric et al. (1991) published two studies of SPECT regarding the obsessive compulsive disorder. In the first of them, ten patients diagnosed with OCD, with eight controls matched by age and sex, found that the blood supply in the medial frontal region of the patients was higher than in the controls, but this did not occur in the orbitofrontal region. They found no correlation between scores on obsession and compulsion scales and blood flow values; and negatively with those of the anxiety scales, in such a way that the higher score on the anxiety scale showed there was less blood flow in the medial frontal area. In the second study of these same authors, they observed in a sample of six patients that cerebral flow was significantly reduced in the mid-frontal region after the administration of fluoxetine at a dose of 80-100 mg/day for three-four months. Hoehn Sane and Cols. (1991) published a case of a patient who, after administration of fluoxetine at a dose of 100 mg, clinically develops a syndrome of frontal hypofunctionality after achieving a marked improvement in obsessive compulsive symptoms. Rubia et al. (1992) published a study in which they analyzed brain flow with Xe-133 gas, SPECT, and with HMPAO in ten male patients and a control group paired with age and sex. In the study with Xe-133 gas, they do not find differences between patients and controls, but a positive relationship between the severity of obsessive and compulsive symptoms and the blood supply (p = 0, 48). In the study with HMPAO, they found that patients had increased uptake of this substance in the orbital cortex bilaterally, in the bilateral high parietodorsal cortex and left posterofrontal cortex. The head of caudate was found significantly lower brain flow values in the patients with OCD than in the controls.

Naveteur et al. (1992) perform a study with SPECT after inhaling Xenon gas in a sample of ten subjects with marked anxious features and ten matched controls, during the presentation of neutral and anxious auditory stimuli. In subjects with notable anxious traits, there was found to be a lower blood flow in which there was also an asymmetry of greater flow on the right side. Adams et al. (1993) studied a sample of eleven by SPECT with HMPAO-TC99m. Patients included met criteria for DSM-III-r for obsessive compulsive disorder and each patient was evaluated with the Yale-Brown scale for obsessions. A nuclear medicine doctor (who was blinded to the diagnosis of the patients) quantified the images obtained. Eight of the eleven patients presented an asymmetric perfusion in the base of the ganglia, six had alterations on the left side.

Electroencephalographic studies in obsessive compulsive disorders

Pacella and Cois (1944) were the first to publish a study with EEG called, "obsessional neuroses." They found alterations in records of twenty-two out of thirty-one patients. In this study, the diagnostic criteria were not standardized, including one of the patients suffered grand mal seizures. In 1979, Flor-Henry et al. found a frontal defect in the dominant hemisphere (left in most cases) in the EEG spectral analysis of a group of obsessive patients; these patients showed decreased performance in the psychometric tests.

Rapoport et al. (1981) examined the EEG of nine adolescents in a state of vigil and in sleep with primary OCD without finding alterations in the first case, but during sleep, found alterations similar to those of depressed patients: REM latency shortened and a decreased total sleep time. The following year, Insel et al. referred to similar results. Jenike and Brotman, in a 1984 study using EEG on twelve patients who met the criteria of DSM-III for OCD, retrospectively reviewed the EEGs performed on patients in the year before the study. In four of the patients, they found alterations: in one of them, slowness of the waves of both temporal regions; in another, paroxysms of high voltage waves in frontotemporal regions; in a third, paroxysms were limited to the right temporal region; and in the last, bilateral frontotemporal slowness. However, we must take into account that in this study, they do not report the medication they were taking or the clinical state during the registration. Ciesielski et al. published two studies, one in 1981 and the other in 1983, in which they analyzed the evoked potential responses of two groups of obsessive patients before the presentation of light stimuli: passively and with a cognitive task during the realization.

In both studies, there were patients who were taking

antidepressant medications. The amplitudes of visual evoked potentials are lower in patients than in controls, and when performing a cognitive task with greater significance. They measured the amplitude of latency with two electrodes located on the parietal regions on both sides respectively. The differences increased according to the complexity of the task, decreasing the amplitude of the waves in patients and increasing in the control group. Kettl and Marks (1986) describe two cases in which an obsessive picture begins after the start of an epilepsy episode. In the first of them, isolated wave-point complexes are found in temporary origin, more frequent on the right side; and in the second, these same complexes appear, but in the left anterior quadrant (it was a male with an IC = 65) and ventricular widening in the CAT scan.

Malloy et al. (1989) examined cortical evoked potentials in a group of eighteen patients with OCD in response to a task (they were asked to press a button or they stopped doing it before an order that appeared on the screen); the amplitude of the P300 wave was significantly lower in the orbitofrontal region when the task to be performed was the inhibition of the motor act by the order of the screen. By comparing the P300 wave evoked by the inhibition task with respect to the realization of the motor act, it was found that it was broader in the frontal areas; what that these authors interpret as an "inhibitory role." Of the eighteen patients, nine were receiving medication, but the authors found no difference between those who were medicated or not. Sloan et al. (1992) published a study in which anticholinergic drugs with central action significantly slowed down the EEG and reduced the coherence of alpha and beta bands, although they do not affect the latency of visual evoked potentials. Hegere and Juckel (1993) studied the dependence of the intensity of evoked auditory potentials as an indicator of central serotonergic function. The amplitude of the Nl-P2 complex depends largely on the serotonergic innervation, in such a way that a preactivation serotonergic tone would mean that, in the presence of more intense stimuli, a greater amplitude would be found in the evoked potentials.

The NI-P2 complex originates in the primary auditory sensory cortex and the authors are capable, with a dipole analysis, of differentiating the contributions of the primary and secondary auditory cortex in its genesis; being that the most marked dependence is in the primary auditory cortex because it is the one that presents an increased serotonergic effect. The amplitude of the NI-P2 complex also presents a dependence on the intensity of the stimulus in the impulsive personality and "seeker of sensations" that various authors have associated with a low serotonergic function.

Kroll et al. (1993) describe a case of a twenty-six-year-old male of who presents with a temporal lobe epilepsy and obsessive compulsive symptomatology; showed an improvement in his symptomatology and in the registration of the encephalogram after a behavioral psychotherapy treatment together with antiepileptic treatment. For these authors, there would be an alteration in the temporal lobe that could influence the obsessive symptomatology. Kuskowski et al. (1993) published a study in which an EEG is performed on thirteen patients that met criteria of DSM-III-r for OCD, that were not receiving medication, and that was not depressed. All the subjects passed the Wechsler Memory Scale, the Eqala of Delayed Logical Memory, and the Delayed Visual Reproduction Test. The quantitative analysis of the EEG showed a decrease in the absolute logarithm of the power in the delta, beta, and beta wave in the right hemisphere. The standardized measures of the hemispheric asymmetry for the beta wave correlated with a worse response in the Scale of Visual Memory, and a better response in the Verbal Memory Scale. The patients with OCD presented a significant alteration in the performance of visuospatial tasks, but not in the verbal memory with respect to the control group. Prichep et al. (1993) studied a group of patients with OCD, divided into two groups according to the typical or atypical clinical presentation.

In the first group, they found an excess in theta wave in the frontal and frontotemporal cortex, while the second, it presented an increase in the alpha wave. Eighty percent of the members of the first group did not respond to the treatment, while 82% of the members of the second group did. Rubia et al. (1993) studied patients with OCD by brain cartography, not finding a significant difference in electroencephalographic activity at rest between the control group and that of obsessive compulsive patients. They also did not observe significant differences in interhemispheric symmetry measurements. However, with the use of the technique of auditory evoked potentials, they found greater amplitude in some components of these acoustic potentials; especially in those potentials also called "endogenous" because they no longer depend on the physical characteristics of the stimulus, but of the brain's response to them. They found that the N100 wave on left frontal regions was significantly increased in the obsessive patients compared to the control group. This wave has been attributed in the literature to the attention that the subject lends to the stimulus that is presented. These authors interpret that the attention that depends on the activity of the frontal lobe is pathologically increased in patients with OCD, which makes them pay exaggerated attention to stimuli that do not deserve it. Another of the late components of the acoustic potential, the P200 wave, is significantly increased in the right parieto-temporal regions in the obsessive patients, always in comparison with the control group, which would imply a hyperfunction of the mesolimbic system, especially frontotemporal connections mediated by dopamine. The administration of a reuptake inhibitor serotonin produces a normalization of brain electrical activity. For these authors, an increase in serotonin (by inhibiting its reuptake) would increase the inhibition that exerts on dopamine, normalizing dopaminergic pathological hyperactivity in these patients.

Biological models of obsessive compulsive disorders

For years, several characteristics of the so-called "obsessional neurosis" have strongly oriented towards the existence of an organic etiopathology in this disorder. These are the possibilities of observing analogous pictures (especially with compulsive and motor symptoms) after psycho-organic injuries; the improvement with the application of drugs with a very specific neurochemical action profile (serotonergic) or even with stereotactic neurosurgery techniques, and the persistence and general refractoriness to the therapeutics of this type of patient. In spite of this, if the collected data on biological factors in depression are compared, anxiety disorders (non-obsessive compulsive) or schizophrenia with those referring to obsessive compulsive disorder, the latter is very reduced. This can be explained by the scarce incidences of these patients. However, they raise very interesting questions and they can also serve as a model (hyper control vs. lack of control, internal vs. external aggressiveness; etc.) against other psychopathological alterations.

Family predisposition

There are genetic studies that support a polygenic-based hereditary participation, although subject to environmental influences. At least 32 pairs of twins have been described concordant and 19 discordant for OCD (Rudin, 1953; Parker, 1964; Marks et al., 1969; Hoaken and Schnurr, 1980), of which 13 pairs of monozygotic twins are safe concordant and seven discordant. Other studies find a high incidence of obsessive traits in families, but not strictly OCD, and consider that studies with twins are not definitive; pointing out that some predisposition for obsessive behavior is inherited, but not for the full development of the disorder (Insel, 1985).

Alteration of neurotransmission: Serotonergic hypothesis

The rise of the serotonergic hypothesis arises from studies that demonstrate the efficacy of Clomipramine, a potent inhibitor of serotonin reuptake in the treatment of OCD, on an observation, originally made twenty years ago (Lopez-Ibor, 1967, 1969). Based on this hypothesis, Yaryura-Tobias (1977) obtains good efficacy in the treatment of OCD using the amino acid precursor, 1-tryptophan, and made spectacular observations in the improvement of obsessive disorders with use of 5-OR-tryptophan associated with inhibitors of peripheral decarboxylase.

These data have been supported by the following investigations that show that other drugs with potent effect on the inhibition of 5-HT reuptake, such as zimeldine (Kahn, 1984), fluvoxamine (Price, 1987) and fluoxetine (Fontaine, 1985), are antiobsessive agents more effective than drugs with less power, and in the reuptake of 5-HT (nortriptyline, imipramine or desipramine) has also failed compared to some effective MAOIs, such as clorgiline (Insel, 1983; Zohar and Insel, 1987). Patients compliant to clomipramine, to which it has been added to the therapeutic regimen of tryptophan or lithium, have an amplifying effect on the response which supports the hypothesis that increasing serotonergic neurotransmission reduces obsessive symptoms (Rasmussen, 1984). To investigate the central serotonergic function, different agents can be used, starting from the evidence of the therapeutic efficacy of the inhibitors of 5-HT reuptake, it could be hypothesized that the administration of a serotonergic agonist to patients with OCD reduced the symptoms; however, a single dose of chlorphenil-piperazine (m-CPP), an agonist of the serotonergic postsynaptic receptor (Mueller et al., 1985), produces a transient but marked exacerbation of the obsessive compulsive symptoms which does not occur in controls or in patients with OCD after placebo (Zohar and collaborators, 1987).

When m-CPP is administered after treatment with clomipramine, obsessive symptoms are not significantly increased; this is consistent with the development of adaptive hyposensitivity of the postsynaptic receptor of 5-Hl to the mCPP agonist after chronic treatment with clomipramine (Zohar, 1988). This data, together with other previous ones that suggest an alteration of the 5-Hl turnover (an increase of 5-HIAA in the LCR, Insel, 1985), direct that some population of 5-HT1 receptors presents hypersensitivity in OCD. The induction of hyposensitivity in these receptors could be the anti-obsessive action mechanism of clomipramine. Charney et al. (1988), in a similar designed work, could not confirm these results. Hemesh et al. (1988) found low levels of vitamin B12 in patients with OCD (20%), significantly higher than in normal and schizophrenic patients (4%), hypothesizing a possible role of vitamin B12 deficiency in pathophysiology of OCD by the interaction between this vitamin and 5-Hl in the CNS, based on the findings of Botez et al. (1982), who found low levels of 5-HIAA in the CSF of neuropsychiatric patients who had deficiencies of vitamin B12 and folate, and who those patients who responded favorably to folate treatment showed an elevation of the 5-HIAA level.

Casas (1986) observed in two patients who had received cyproterone acetate (drug; antiandrogen); one of them for the treatment of hirsutism and another that initiated a process of feminization, through the improvement of obsessive symptoms. Based on this finding, he initiated a pilot study of treatment with cyproterone acetate to six women with OCD resistant to treatment with anxiolytics and antidepressants. He observed improvement of symptoms during the pharmacological treatment with reappearance after the withdrawal of the drug. There are findings that support the hypothesis that gonadal hormones are important in the development of serotonergic systems. So it has been seen that gonadectomy in rats determined an increase in SHT levels on day 12 if the animals were males, and levels frankly inferior to those of this group if they were females. On the other hand, administration of estradiol or diethylstilbestrol in rats at birth determined an increase of 5-HT in both sexes detectable on days 8 and 12 (Essman, 1978). Testosterone could exert an enzymatic effect, thereby reducing the concentration of SHT in males or maybe estrogens acts directly on the brain tissue increasing its capacity to produce 5-HT in the neonatal female.

Dopaminergic hypothesis

The anti-obsessive action of periciazine is an example of the possible therapeutic effectiveness of dopaminergic block. It is also indicated for OCD with a set of nosological entities presumably linked to an alteration of the dopaminergic neurotransmission system, such as schizophrenia, tardive dyskinesia, Huntington's chorea, and, above all, the syndrome of Gilles de la Tourette. In some of these disorders, the frequency of onset of obsessive compulsive symptoms becomes the same as in the case of the syndrome of Gilles de la Tourette - from 33 to 89 years old, according to the authors (Turner, 1985; 1984). Even the possibility of a common genetics for both disorders, it is suggested by Pauls and Leckman (1986) that OCD can be represented as an alternative expression for the factors responsible for Gilles de la Tourette syndrome. There are compulsive stereotyped behaviors in amphetamine psychosis and the utility of haloperidol (dopamine receptor blocker) in the treatment of Tourette which have led to present OCD symptoms as the result of hyperactivity.

Catecholaminergic hypothesis

The administration of clonidine has been found to dull the growth hormone (GH) in OCD patients (Siever, 1983; Insel, 1984) as in patients with melancholy. This test assesses the function of the adrenergic receptor. In normal conditions, administration of clonidine agonist determines an increase in plasma GH, probably by a direct postsynaptic effect on hypothalamic receptors. The decrease in this response would imply a decrease in reflex adrenergic activity of a lower sensitivity of central adrenergic receptors. Siever (1983), consistent with this hypothesis, found higher MHPG plasma levels in patients with OCD than in controls, which suggests the possibility that in these patients, there could be an increase in presynaptic noradrenergic activity and a compensatory decrease of postsynaptic adrenergic receptors.

Endorphinic hypothesis

Insel and Pickar (1983) hypothesized that obsessive patients with ruminative doubts had a deficit, mediated by opiates, in the ability to record the reward; this deficit could manifest itself at the cognitive level as a difficulty in reaching certainty. These authors found that the administration of naloxone to two patients with OCD had a worsening of acute symptoms, which did not occur after placebo. Clomipramine has been shown to improve obsessive symptoms; it has also been proven its antinociceptive actions of opiates (Sewel and Lee, 1980). In addition, d-amphetamine causes brief but significant improvement in patients with severe obsessions (Insel et al. Cols., 1983). This effect of d-amphetamine may be related to the opiate system since naloxone blocks the increase in activation and self-stimulation caused by the d-amphetamine (Segal et al., 1979). These findings imply opioids in some way are endogenous in the pathophysiology of the obsessive symptom.

Organic brain damage

The association of OCD with brain damage: In 1963, Schilder speculated for the first time the possible organic etiology of the disorder when observing the association between OCD and encephalitis, and when finding neurological abnormalities in several patients, such as moderate tremor, decreased movement of the arms, rigid faces, akinesia and hyperkinesia. Mayer-Gross (1960) describes it as a common sequela of encephalitis, Parkinson's disease, and cranial trauma. Barton (1954, 1965) describes a patient with OCD who had diabetes insipidus, speculating that the disorder could be secondary to hypothalamic alteration. Hillbom (1960), in a review of 414 cases of cranial traumatisms of war found a prevalence of obsessive neurosis of 3.4%; however Lishman (1968) only observed the development of the disorder in 1.4% of those who presented severe head trauma, concluding that it could be an infrequent variety of post-traumatic sequelae. Four cases of OCD have recently been described whose onset was preceded by mild head trauma (McKeon et al., 1984) and whose symptoms began within twenty-four hours after the trauma.

In general, the engine components of OCD (stereotypes, compulsions) predominate over these patients. Behar (1984), using the CT, reports a cerebral ventricular dilation significantly higher in adolescents with OCD than in controls, as well as deficits perceptual-spatial similar to those found in patients with lesions of the lobule temporary. Behar himself points out the possibility that the group of subjects with OCD beginning in childhood constitutes a subgroup with more marked CNS dysfunction. A psychophysiological technique to investigate if there is any altered brain information process is the study of evoked potentials. Thus, Ciesielki (1981) and Beech (1983) demonstrate on the N220 wave of visually evoked potentials, a decrease in amplitude and a shortening of its latency similar to those that occur to psychotic patients, which could mean a disorder in the early stages of information processing complex, for lack of inhibitory control. Ciesielski comments that the shortening of the latency is compatible with the hypothesis of a deficit of 5-HT neurotransmitter system of primarily inhibitor type. Shagass (1984) studies the evoked potentials somatosensory in patients with OCD, schizophrenia, and major depression, finding characteristically in patients with OCD, that the average amplitude of the N60 was greater (more negative), while that of P90 tended to be smaller (less positive, also the amplitude of wave N130 was also lower, less negative). Shagass thinks that of confirming these results, somatosensory evoked potentials could be used for the differential diagnosis of OCD. Among the slow potentials, the contingent negative variation (CNV) does not provide significant data regarding the morphology and resolution of the wave but demonstrates a decrease in its amplitude (Valliejo, 1979) that can be interpreted in terms of the high level of activation or as an alteration of attention processes. It is also common to find alterations in neuropsychological tests in these patients. Sher et al. (1984) proved that there is a memory deficit with regard to daily activities in compulsive patients with checking rituals, but not in the rest of the patients with OCD. Naturally, the decrease in attention concentration could explain the finding.

Improvement after neurosurgery

Bernstein et al. (1975) show the follow-up of 43 psychiatric patients whom he had practiced a prefrontal lobotomy between 1948 and 1970, finding that OCD (N = 27) improved more than schizophrenic patients. After reviewing the catamnesis of leucotomies performed since 1941 (about 80 sick), they proved to have surprisingly long-term results (Peraita and Cois, 1972). The leucotomy is based on the disconnection of the frontothalamic pathways as has a favorable effect on the patient's emotional cognition. In 1947, Spiegel and Wycis introduce the stereotactic technique which allows a greater precision and safety by limiting injuries to more specific areas. In 1952, some researchers (Whitty and Colabs., 1952; Le Beau, 1952) found that lesions in the cingulo-opercular network did not cause any change in psychotic, but relieved the obsessive and anxious states. Gray-Walter (1977) theorized that over-activation of the cingulate caused compulsive bingeing; Talairach and Colabs (1973) verified the production of similar repetitive stereotyped movements to the compulsive rituals induced by the electrical stimulation of the cingular region in 52 epileptic patients resistant to treatments. Mitchel-Heggs et al. (1976) observed that surgery, consisting of two small lesions in the medial quadrant of each frontal lobe, led to a definite clinical improvement in 89% of 27 severely obsessive patients. Leksell developed the bilateral stereotactic anterior capsulotomy technique, whose better results are focused on obsessive patients (Fodstad et al., 1982) and are comparable to those obtained with the cingulotomy. Among those, López-Ibor et al. (1973) reviewed 24 operative cases with the technique of stereotactic capsulotomy, and observed that in 80% of the patients, hyperthymic phases appeared in the first week of the postoperative period, or in any case, before six months, coinciding with the normalization of the state of mind with the disappearance or attenuation of phobic and obsessive phenomena to stop the symptoms from being a burden for the psychic life of the patients. Tippin and Henn (1982) found that five severely obsessive patients, there was an improvement (one of which with complete remission) after modified leucotomy with the elimination of 2-3 medial centimeters of the white substance that goes from the anterior cingulate gyrus.

This procedure is thought to act by interrupting the

thalamus-frontal tract. Burzaco (1980) has made an exhaustion review of the subjects, relying on a broad personal experience (85 obsessive patients operated on until 1981). The area of incidence of stereotactic psychosurgery focuses on diencephalic connections (tractotomy suborbital, anterior capsulotomy, cingulotomy, medial thalamotomy). Severe patients far exceeded 50% improvement! The most specific operative fields in these patients seem to definitely focus on the subcaudate and cingulate areas.

Co-morbidity in obsessive compulsive disorders

Often, obsessive compulsive disorder is associated with other pathologies, of which major depression and anxiety disorders are the most frequent. Rasmussen and Bisen, in 1992, published a study in which they found that patients with OCD have the probability of suffering depression throughout their life, using the Schedule for Affective Disorder and the Schizophrenic Lifestyle Anxiety (SADS) of 78%.

The presence of phobias is frequent within OCD with a

SADS = 28%; separation anxiety of a 17%. The probability of presenting a social phobia throughout the life of an individual with OCD is of a SADS = 26%, while the probability of suffering an eating disorder is SADS = 8%, alcohol abuse, and panic disorders are also frequently associated with this disorder (SADS = 16% and SADS = 15%, respectively). The probability of suffering a motor disorder, especially the Gilles de la Tourette Syndrome, is also higher than expected by chance, with a SADS = 6%.

However, not all disorders that receive the "compulsive" qualification form part of the obsessive compulsive disorder. Many disorders such as kleptomania, pyromania, trichotillomania, "compulsive shopping," and gambling, have the repetitive behavior in common with OCD. Most of them are due to lack of impulse control, although there is data in favor of a serotonergic dysfunction involved in its etiopathogenesis. Rieman et al. (1992) found an interesting association: the rate of alcoholism among patients with OCD is not superior to the normal population, however, alcoholics have rates of OCD superior to the general population. In 1993, Crum et al. used data from the Epidemiologic Catchment Area Investigation (ECA) to study whether the incidence of OCD was superior in consumers of illicit drugs. The sample consisted of 13,306 people, of which 414 were habitual users of cocaine. They found that subjects who used cocaine and other drugs such as marijuana, had a higher risk of developing OCD; this risk was estimated at 7.1% ($p = 0.03$) for the consuming subjects versus 4.1% ($p = 0.01$) in the population that did not consume drugs.

OCD has been linked on occasion to post-traumatic stress disorder. Recent epidemiological studies find much higher rates of OCD among veterans of the Vietnam War than in the general population. Pitman and Cols (1993) describe a case of an individual who did not suffer from any psychopathology before the war, yet had OCD accompanied by post-traumatic stress disorder after, and whose symptoms persisted for more than twenty years. The use of cosmetic surgery in patients with dysmorphobia remains controversial, although, in the short term, it is beneficial. Jerone et al. (1992) published a controlled study of 20 patients who were on the waiting list for an aesthetic operation of rhinoplasty in comparison with a control group. In terms of psychiatric mortality, patients who presented with more alterations (than controls) had high rates of neuroticism, social phobia and were much less extroverted. In terms of body image, results suggest that those who were on the waiting list met some of the essential criteria of dysmorphobia. Lydiar et al (1993) find that dysmorphobia has common characteristics with obsessive compulsive disorder and social phobia; in fact, in Japanese and Korean literature, it is considered a form of social phobia. However, it is known that social phobia that presents in these patients is usually secondary to dysmorphophobic disorder. These authors have also noticed a response to the different treatment since dysmorphobia responds primarily to SSRIs, while social phobia responds to SSRIs but also to MAOIs.

Philips et al. (1994) found that 9 (19%) of patients with OCD had dysmorphobia, but that none of them had mentioned it to a doctor because it was very embarrassing. It is very important to identify this disorder since it has a high rate of suicide attempts and also has a good response to treatment. They differ from Jerone (1992) who thinks that patients with dysmorphobia respond spectacularly to surgical treatment because they argue that these rarely produce a satisfactory response, and even in many cases produce a deterioration of the symptomatology. "Compulsive shopping" has been ignored for a long time in the psychiatric literature although it is apparently frequent and can cause severe consequences both from the economic point of view and legal. Schlosser et al. (1994) designed a study to assess the lifestyle and problems of 'compulsive buyers.' Forty-six patients were studied with the structured interview of the DSM-III-r for disorders of personality and with a semi-structured interview focused on this disorder. The profile was that of a 31-year-old woman who started at age 18. These subjects spend their money on clothes, shoes, and music. More than two-thirds met criteria for a disorder (axis I); the most frequent were anxiety disorders, substance abuse, and disorders of humor. Almost 60% met criteria for personality disorder (axis II), more often they were obsessive compulsive, borderline, or by avoidance. For these authors, it is a clinical entity that can cause a large discomfort to those who suffer from it and it is also associated with other disorders psychiatric. The relationship of obsessive compulsive disorder has also been studied with psychotic disorders. Elsen et al. (1993) studied of a total of 475 patients undergoing ambulatory treatment for OCD; 67 (14%) had psychotic symptoms which were defined as hallucinations, delirious ideas, and thought disorders. For 6% of the sample, it was the little bit of introspection. Four percent of patients met DSM-III-r criteria for both OCD and schizophrenia, and 3% met criteria for schizotypal disorder of the personality.

Co-morbidity with eating disorders

Since 1939, a large number of authors have found common characteristics in different morbid processes that, according to the DSM-III-r classification, are known as obsessive compulsive disorder, eating disorders, and mood disorders. Du Bois, in 1949, grouped these common characteristics according to phenomenological aspects, response to treatment, and family history. The obsessive fear of gaining weight, rituals in diets, and a strict schedule of meals are all common events in patients with anorexia nervosa and may be related to obsessive compulsions (Palmer et al., 1939; Solyom et al., 1982) which are typical of OCD. "Obsessive guilt" feelings appear in bulimic patients when they eat disproportionately and the habit of provoking vomit shows psychopathological relationships with obsessions and compulsions (Solyom et al., 1982). There are common symptoms of OCD, eating, and mood disorders, such as, for example, decreased interest in sex, a decrease in body temperature, and sleep inhibition. Fahy et al. (1993) studied a sample of 105 women with OCD, of which twelve women (11%) had a history of anorexia nervosa. Some patients initially presented with obsessive compulsive symptoms; while in patients suffering from OCD together with anorexia nervosa, the symptomatology appeared at the same time. The co-morbidity between these two syndromes seems to be related to common vulnerability factors. Patients in whom OCD appears at an early age have an increased risk of developing disorders of alimentary behavior. For Iancu et al. (1993), there would be socio-cultural factors involved in the pathogenesis of anorexia nervosa with a clinical relationship between eating disorders, depression, and OCD. They presented a case of a sixteen-year-old woman, an immigrant from Russia, that develops the three pathologies. Tamburrino et al. (1994) published a study in which they examined the frequency of eating disorders in women with OCD. All patients were passed through the Yale-Brown scale for obsessions and compulsions. Thirty-one women participated in the study, of which 42% (n = 13) had a history of behavior disorders of food - 26% anorexia nervosa (n = 8); 3% bulimia nervosa (n = 1); and 13% anorexia and bulimia (n = 4). These authors consider that the frequency of an eating disorder to develop before developing OCD is superior; this is still believed until now. Pascuale et al. (1994)

calculate the morbidity rate in families of patients with eating disorders (n = 41), obsessive compulsive disorder (n = t70), and humor disorder (n = 39). The family risk for developing obsessive compulsive disorder was higher in those families that already had a history of OCD. Also, there was a statistically significant association in families with antecedents of eating and mood disorders.

Co-morbidity with alterations of the central nervous system

Throughout history, various themes have been formulated around the etiology of the obsessive compulsive disorder and the idea that OCD could be related to an organic cerebral disturbance. This was exposed by Tuke at the end of the 19th century, who argued that the symptoms of the disorder were often present in the von Economo encephalitis and in temporal lobe epilepsy. However, it is not until recent times when it has been possible to systematize studies that provide results in favor of this hypothesis. Currently, there is data that supports that OCD may appear in association with certain conditions which are known to alter the function of the nervous system, while in other cases it is possible to identify relevant neurological history in the personal history of the patient with this disorder.

In the same way, the response to pharmacotherapy and evaluation of the nervous system through neurophysiological techniques and imaging, and through neuropsychological studies, demonstrates the existence of diverse alterations in these patients, which also indicates a commitment in the operation of specific brain areas. These facts have led to the development of neurobiological models of OCD based on anatomical concepts. Models that develop from anatomical concepts focus their attention on the symptomatology of OCD in other neurological diseases, whose neurophysiopathogenic mechanisms are known or at least can be documented with paraclinical techniques. Within this line of research, it is hypothesized that the basal ganglia and frontal cortex play a decisive role in the pathophysiology of OCD. Another support for neurobiological models from anatomical concepts is constituted by the fact that the obsessive compulsive symptomatology can appear after cranioencephalic trauma because, in some extreme cases, it can be treated surgically. Within these studies, particular attention is paid to the participation of temporal, frontal and other areas of the cerebral cortex in the obsessive compulsive symptoms.

On the other hand, advances in genetic engineering have led to the development of diverse techniques that allow us to evaluate from an anatomical and physiological point of view the conditions of the central nervous system. The alterations in the frontal-subcortical systems have been related to the pathogenesis of OCD. On the other hand, there are relationships between OCD and other neurological disorders such as Gilles de la Tourette syndrome, neuroacanthosis, postencephalitic parkinsonism, caudate nucleus infarction, monoxide poisoning carbon, manganese poisoning, anoxia, progressive supranuclear paralysis, chorea Sydenham, and lesions in the frontal lobe. All this indicates that the palecaudado frontal circuit means the symptomatology of OCD and Gilles de la Tourette syndrome is defined as the chronic presence of motor and verbal tics. Erenberg et al (1987) published a study on the natural evolution of tics in an adult population of 58 subjects, aged between 15 and 25 years. They found that tics "almost disappeared" in 26% or at least decreased by 47%. Fourteen percent remained unchanged and symptoms worsened in another 14%. In addition, they found that 41% of patients older than 18 years should continue receiving medication. In 1988, Brun studied a sample of 136 patients with Tourette syndrome between the ages of 5 and 15 years old, finding that the severity of the symptoms improved over time; 28% were able to do without the medication and 52% of the cases had spontaneous improvements. Shapiro, in 1989, found that 5 to 8% of patients with this disorder recovered completely and this recovery remained in adolescence; the tics were less severe in 35% of the cases during adolescence and less severe in almost all adult patients.

There is recent evidence that specific behavioral

disorders, including obsessive compulsive disorder and attention deficit with hyperkinesia, are associated with a frequency higher than expected to develop or also be diagnosed with Gilles syndrome of the Tourette. Several studies show that from 30 to 50% of patients with Tourette's syndrome also has obsessive compulsive disorder. Studies in families demonstrate that the etiology of the two disorders is related. In a study published by Leonard (1992), results found that 54 children and adolescents with severe, primary OCD with tics but that did not meet Gilles criteria, were reassessed at 2-7 years and diagnosed with Gilles de la Tourette syndrome. So the question becomes- does OCD also have tics? Structured interviews and exams were used for neurological testing to determine the presence of tics in these patients and in 171 relatives of the first degree. A family history of tics was found in 57% of patients at beginning of the study, while at the end of the follow-up it increased up to 59%. Eight patients met criteria for Tourette syndrome. Patients with a history family of tics showed great anxiety, an increased concentration of 5-

OHindoleacetic acid and homovallinic acid; they also presented as OCD of earlier appearance.

Patients with Gilles only differed in the age of onset of OCD. The frequency of the appearance of the Tourette syndrome and tics among first-degree relatives was 1.8% and 14% respectively. This study is the first to be systematized and supports the hypothesis that OCD and Gilles de la Tourette syndrome can be manifestations of the same genetic disease. Park et al., in 1993, published a retrospective study on a sample of 101 children with Tourette's syndrome which were characterized by an early onset of disease and were also associated with behavioral disorders- attention deficit by hyperkinesia (45%), obsessive compulsive disorder (50%), highly disturbed behavior (67%) and school problems (52%). Of the patients who presented alterations of behavior at the beginning of the table, those that improved at the end of treatment included 46% of those who had attention deficit disorder with hyperkinesia, 47% of those who presented OCD, 46% of those who had a very altered behavior and 66% of those who had school problems. The follow-up of the patients was carried out every 6 months. At the end of the study, those that needed treatment for tics was 10%, anti-obsessive treatment was 5% and those that needed stimulants was 12%; significantly decreased from the beginning.

Pauls et al., in 1993, published a paper with a sample of 338 first-degree relatives of 85 patients with Gilles de la Tourette syndrome and 113 controls. They used structured interviews and family history collected from each member. They found no evidence that attention disorders, learning problems, stuttering, and language problems were variants of the syndrome of Tourette. These authors believe that there would be two types of attention deficit disorders in relationship with Gilles; one would be a secondary form to the latter and in the other, the association would be casual. Robertson et al (1993) examined the relationship between obsessive compulsive disorder and Tourette syndrome; compare to obsessive, depressive, and anxiety symptoms in a group of patients with Gilles with a group of depressed patients and with a control group. The score on *obsession* scales was higher in the first group and in the group of depressed than in control subjects. The score on *depression* scales was also higher in the first group than in the control subjects but much lower than in the depressed subjects. These findings suggest that patients with Gilles have a high probability of presenting with primary OCD and also to develop obsessive compulsive symptoms when they get depressed.

Although OCD often occurs in patients with Gilles syndrome of the Tourette, little is known about the characteristics that present in these patients and, if these differ or not from those that appear in those they have a pure OCD. Mark et al. (1993) develop a prospective study with a sample of 10 subjects and 15 subjects with OCD and Tourette syndrome respectively. They used as measuring instruments the Yak-Brown scale for obsessions and compulsions, the questionnaire of Leyton obsessions, and a questionnaire designed to differentiate the symptoms between both groups.

The subjects who presented OCD associated with the syndrome the Tourette had statistically significantly higher obsessions on violent subjects, sexual, and symmetry needs. In the subjects that suffered the two pathologies, the compulsions appeared spontaneously while in subjects suffering from pure OCD were preceded by obsessions. Therefore, these authors find that OCD and the syndrome of Gilles de la Tourette associated with OCD have phenomenological differences and believe that they could correspond to the existence of differences in neuroanatomical or neurochemical connections.

These same authors (Mark et al., 1993) carried out a study in which they compared the relationship between 5-HT and dopamine in both disorders for 14 weeks and double-blinded; this study compared fluvoxamine (a selective inhibitor of the reuptake of serotonin) with sulpiride (an antagonist of the dopamine D2 receptors), and was followed by a single-blinded study with combination therapy (4 weeks) in 11 subjects who presented OCD and Gilles de la Tourette. Sulpiride reduced tics but did not improve the obsessive compulsive symptoms; Fluvoxamine alone or combined with sulpiride did not improve tics but instead, it reduced the obsessive symptomatology. It is possible that the dopaminergic pathways and serotoninergic agents are implicated in this disorder. The presence of OCD in patients with Huntington's disease, a disease autosomal dominant neurodegenerative disorder characterized by choreiform movements and progressive dementia, has been found in some cases. Cummings et al. (1992) published a study with two cases; both patients showed repetitive behaviors and characteristics of OCD. Possibly, the frontal-caudate-pale circuit plays an important role in the onset of symptoms of OCD.

Cognitive deficits in patients with structural lesions of the basal ganglia usually include a decrease in verbal fluency, a slowness, difficulty in the ambition of tasks, a decrease in spatial orientation, and a difficulty in learning motor tasks. Martin et al. (1993) conducted a study proposed to determine if patients with OCD had those same cognitive dysfunctions. A battery of neuropsychological tests was given to a sample of 17 patients with OCD (not on treatment) and to 16 controls that matched in age and sex. Eleven patients were also evaluated with trichotillomania. Their results suggest that the brain regions responsible for the cognitive dysfunctions in patients with Huntington's disease are different than those involved in OCD. Idiopathic spasmodic torticollis, due to an alteration of the basal ganglia, is a form of cervical dystonia characterized by involuntary movements of the muscles of the neck that causes a clonic deviation of the head or the adoption of abnormal postures. Bihari et al. (1992) studied the relationship between obsessive compulsive symptoms of 22 patients with spasmodic torticollis and 29 controls. Using the Yale-Brown scales for obsessions and compulsions, the Maudsley questionnaire for obsessions and compulsions, and the Beck depression questionnaire, they found that subjects with torticollis spasmodic symptoms had more obsessive compulsive symptoms, depression, and anxiety than control subjects. Blepharospasm, a disorder characterized by involuntary orbicular muscle contractions that causes a continuous flicker or involuntary closing of the eyelids, is a form of focal dystonia, which shares phenomenological characteristics with OCD. To evaluate this relationship, Bihari et al. (1992) used the Maudsley questionnaire for obsessions and compulsions on a sample population of 21 patients with biefrospasm and 19 control subjects. The cases obtained higher scores than controls.

Swedo et al. (1993) studied 11 children with Sydenham chorea with a clinic that included dysarthria, gait disorders, and involuntary movements of the face, neck, trunk, and extremities. Ten of the 11 children had antineuronal antibodies and all had psychological alterations; especially obsessive compulsive symptoms, emotional lability, hyperactivity, irritability, distractibility, and more childish behavior. The obsessive compulsive symptoms appeared in 9 children (82%) of which 4 met DSM-III-r criteria for OCD. Trichotillomania is classified within the DSM-III-r as a control disorder of impulses, although it has phenomenological characteristics that respond to treatment, and common family and neurobiological associations with OCD. Leane et al. (1992), in a family study, found that the relationship between OCD and trichotillomania is 94%. A sample of 65 first-degree relatives of 16 women with chronic trichotillomania was compared with two control groups. The first was formed by 90 first-class relatives of 19 healthy volunteer women matched in age, and the other group consisted of 65 normal controls. Of the 16 women with trichotillomania, 19% had first-degree relatives with obsessive compulsive disorder. Three of the 65 relatives were diagnosed with OCD. In the family of the healthy women group, no family member met criteria for OCD. These results show an elevated rate of OCD in relatives of patients with trichotillomania.

Swann et al (1992) compared 8 patients with trichotillomania with 13 patients with OCD. For these authors, there are differences in the symptomatology since individuals with trichotillomania get more pleasure when they pull their hair than individuals with OCD when they perform their rituals. Patients with trichotillomania have less anxiety, depression, neurosis, and are more extroverted. Hunt (1993) published a case of a woman with trichotillomania who did not respond to treatment with clomipramine, fluoxetine or buspirone, but which improved with trazodone. Each case suggests that trichotillomania symptoms respond favorably to trazodone, especially if it is associated with obsessive compulsive symptoms such as this case.

Co-morbidity with depressive states

The psychopathological relationship between obsessive compulsive disorder and mood disorders has been studied for a long time. Krafft-Ebing highlighted the identity of obsessive and melancholic thoughts; and Kraepelin, Maudsley, and Marchand considered that obsessions were an integral part or at least very related to the disorders of the humor, especially with melancholic episodes. Currently and following Freud's psychodynamic theory, obsessive compulsive disorder is classified within anxiety disorders as can be seen in the

Diagnostic and Statistical Manual of the American Psychiatric Association (DSM-I) (APA, 1952), in the DSM-II (APA, 1969), and in the ninth edition of the International Classification of Diseases of the World Health Organization (ICD-9) (WHO, 1987). However, clinical observations made during the 1960s suggest, for the first time once again, the possibility that this supposed unitary nosological category is based, in reality, in entities with different etiological and clinical points of view. The DSM-III (APA, 1980) proposed a reclassification of anxiety disorders- the term "neurosis" is abandoned because it implies the fact of sharing a common cause; a conflict of the unconscious related to an inadequate use of the defense mechanisms of the individual. Instead of considering the etiology of the morbid process, the DSM-1II classification is based on the presence of common symptoms.

The multiaxial system was established to separately assess personality disorders, possible organic etiologies, environmental stresses, and levels of adaptation prior to clinical manifestations. As a consequence of this, the compulsive personality presents on axis II, clearly separated from obsessive compulsive disorder on axis I. One of the most controversial aspects of anxiety disorders, in general, is the autonomy or independence of mood disorders. This has caused the appearance of opposing views, advocates of separation into different categories (Roth et al. 1972), and those that support the unitary hypothesis of affective and emotional disorders. For example, Lewis (1934) found high prevalence rates of panic attacks and OCD in melancholic patients. Even before Lewis, Janet (1903) maintained the clinical unity of the forced agitations, a set of disorders that included obsessive disorders, panic, phobias, bulimia, syndromes with pain (including some cases of migraine and atypical facial pain), and other psychological disorders such as irritable bowel syndrome. Janet found that the forced agitations were frequently associated with dysthymia and depression (psychasthenic and neurasthenia respectively).

Lopez Ibor (1950-1966) described the "vital anguish" as the cardinal symptom of neurotic disorders, which was an anguish of a biological nature (endotimic). The vital anguish was analogous to the "vital sadness" described by Schneider (1950) in depression. However, neurotic disorders were not confused with other mood disorders. being one of the types or subcategories. In addition, Lopez's investigations were more related to etiopathogenesis and psychopathology than with nosology; he also proposed biological treatments for neurotic conditions. For the diagnosis of OCD, the DSM-III requires that obsessions and compulsions not be secondary to another mental disorder, such as the Gilles syndrome of the Tourette, schizophrenia, major depression, or organic mental disorder. However, in the revised version DSM-III-r (APA, 1987), these exclusion criteria were eliminated because it was recognized that OCD could appear along with other disorders. Some authors propose the phrase "with psychotic symptoms" for severe cases of OCD, that just like in mood disorders, they have intrusive thoughts that acquire the quality of delusion and to which the individual does not offer resistance.

In the ICD-10, OCD is separated from other neurotic

disorders, confirming what is in concordance with recent investigations; that is, the consideration of OCD as an independent entity. At the same time, OCD is a heterogeneous condition with different stages in its evolution and perhaps clinical subforms. The different stadiums of OCD were, for the first time, described by Legrand du Saulle (1875), and admitted later by Janet (1903).

Clinical Manifestations

There is enough data in favor of the possible association between OCD and mood disorders (Insel et al., 1982a, 1984), consequently, are frequently adjoined in investigations looking into the relationships of obsessions, compulsions, and depression (Gittelson, 1966; Welner et al 1976; Videbach, 1975). This topic can be considered from different perspectives. Depressive symptoms in obsessive compulsive disorder are not uncommon for patients with OCD; they simultaneously present with all symptoms (Jenike et al 1981, 1990, 1991). Rasmussen and Tsuang, in a sample of 100 patients diagnosed with OCD, found that up to 20% denied having depression at the beginning of the study and most referred that depression had appeared after the onset of obsessive compulsive symptoms. A minority presented obsessive and depressive symptoms at the same time. From Rosenberg (1968), up to 34% of patients with OCD had previously received antidepressant treatment. During the depressive episode, the obsessive symptoms increased in some patients but decreased in others.

On the other hand, many patients with OCD only go to the doctor when they get depressed. This would increase the prevalence of depression in these clinical studies. Kringlen found than 17% of patients with OCD had depressive symptoms at the beginning of their symptomatology, but 42% had these symptoms at the time of hospitalization.

Obsessions and compulsions in depressive disorder

Obsessions and compulsions are frequent in primary mood disorders (Zohar and Insel, 1987a). In fact, some have pointed out that depression with obsessive compulsive symptoms represents a subtype of mood disorders. Obsessive symptoms may appear during a major depressive episode, usually related to depressive symptomatology such as obsessive thoughts of doubt. It is described that obsessions reduce the risk of suicide in the depressive (Jenike, 1991). In a retrospective study of 398 depressive patients with psychotic features, Gittleson (1966) found that 152 (38%) had obsessive symptoms. In these patients, the presence of obsessions was related to previous depressive personality traits. This author also found that depressed patients with obsessive features had fewer suicidal attempts than those who did not have obsessive characteristics. However, Videbach (1975) could not verify this protective effect of the obsessions on suicide; later this author and Vaughan (1966) found that the obsessive traits were more fervent in agitated depressions than in inhibited ones.

The course of obsessions and compulsions seems to be parallel to the primary disorder (OCD). The obsessive symptoms tend to appear during depression and decrease as the patient improves; if the obsessive symptoms commence earlier, they get worse during depression and then they return to the original state at the moment when the depressive episode ceases (Videbach, 1975; Marks, 1987).

Similarities and differences between depressive and obsessive symptoms

There are many common symptoms of both disorders which makes it difficult to separate OCD from OCD of depression. In both disorders, there is low self-esteem, feelings of doubt, anxiety, and guilt. The vegetative symptoms, such as weight loss and sleep disturbances, can also appear in OCD; the rituals related to food intake and sleep are frequent during a depressive episode. It is also difficult to differentiate concerns of a depressive personality to the obsessive thoughts that appear in OCD. Generally, the ruminations are egosyntonic, meaning they are accepted by the patient's rational, perhaps exaggerated but related to the depressive experience. However, the obsessions are egodystonic and are experienced by the subject as imposed, out of context, and to which the subject offers resistance. While the depressed patient tends to focus everything in the past, the obsessive patient tends to prevent future events.

Aggression is a common phenomenon in OCD and in depression, but this symptom is different. Depressed patients always show poor control of their aggressiveness especially at the beginning and end of an episode (Ledesma, 1977), while patients with OCD are good controllers; very rarely do they lose control, but when it happens, they tend to be very violent. Vulnerability to depression is characterized by excessive adaptation to social norms, but patients with OCD are characterized because, on the one hand, they seem to adapt extraordinarily well to the social norms since they are very perfectionist, but when the activity becomes ritualistic, it loses its meaning. So for example, the ritual of washing does not translate into cleanliness, yet moral obsessions cause the individual to have a moral behavior.

Clinical course

The course of both diseases is different. Depression tends to be processed via episodes while OCD is chronic (Coryell, 198 1). The age of appearance of OCD is comparatively lower than depression, and the male/female relationship is also different (lower for depression). Kendell and Discipio (1970) observed that obsessive symptoms are rare in mania. The disappearance of obsessive compulsive symptoms has been described in OCD and in bipolar disorder during manic episodes, (Gordon and Rasmussen, 1988). Another interesting fact is that depressive symptoms improve with pregnancy while obsessions get worse (Brandt and Mackenzie, 1987).

Family studies

Both depression and OCD tend to appear in the same families, suggesting the possible existence of an association between these diseases, although the nature of this association is not yet clear. In a retrospective study, Coryell (1981) found that obsessive patients had a high frequency of family history of mania or depression compared to the control group (20.9% versus to 4.6%).

Epidemiology

There is also an association of these two diseases in the general population. Boyd et al. (1984) found that using a multiple diagnostic systems in patients with OCD, they had a probability of 10.8 superior to suffer depression than individuals who did not suffer from this disorder. Obsessive and depressive symptoms sometimes appear frequently at the same time in a patient. In the USA, the ECA study found that one-third of obsessive patients met DSM-III-r criteria for major depression. Because of this, it seems that depression is the most frequent complication of OCD. It can appear before, during, or after the obsessive symptoms and can follow an independent course or not (Marks et al, 1975).

Secondary depression in OCD; Comorbidity between both disorders

In many patients with OCD, depressive episodes remain after a long time of obsessive disorder. This causes clinicians to tend to diagnose OCD when the depressive symptoms appear later. According to this theory, the basic disorder is the primary, and the secondary derives from it. When depressive symptoms appear with priority, the prognosis is better. The chronological sequence of depression and obsession seems to have a theoretical importance and a utility in clinical practice.

Response to treatment

The response to pharmacological treatment has been used to identify disorders that share a common psychopathology. Some antidepressants (Tricyclics and MAOIs) have demonstrated their efficacy in OCD; however, this disorder does not respond to electroconvulsive therapy (Lieberman, 1984). The fact that inhibitors of serotonin reuptake are effective in OCD while the noradrenaline reuptake inhibitors are not, different from other mood and anxiety disorders. This allows us to raise the hypothesis of a

Effects of Serotonin and Dopamine in Obsessive Compulsive Disorder

possible serotonin dysfunction in OCD. The new selective inhibitors of the reuptake of Serotonin (SSRI) (such as fluoxetine, fluvoxamine, and to a lesser extent mianserin, and other non-tricyclic antidepressants) have been shown to have anti-obsessive effects. In cases of poor response to these treatments, strategies have been developed aimed at increasing the serotoninergic power of the treatments. Depressive symptoms of OCD improve in parallel with the obsessions and compulsions (Flament et al 1985, Perse et al 1987, Cottraux et al 1990, and Godman and Cabbage. 1989); although other studies have not found this parallelism (Ananth et al., 1981, Insel et al. 1983). Another fact that differentiates OCD of depressive disorder is the poor response to placebo observed in OCD. For example, in the Montgomery study (1980), they responded to placebo- 5% of patients, while 65% responded to clomipramine. However, placebo response for depression has greater than 30% reaction. The depressive symptoms that appear in OCD do not respond to placebo. It seems that the mechanism of the action of selective serotonin reuptake inhibitors requires a period of adaptation for the receptors so that the antidepressant effects take place; while in the case of the depression that is part of OCD, this effect could take place more quickly. Sleep deprivation usually produces a short response in half of the depressed patients (Joffe and Brown, 1984). Patients suffering from OCD generally do not respond to sleep deprivation, and their obsessions or compulsions do not change (Joffe and Swinson, 1988).

Thoren et al. (1980) observed that the reduction of 5-HIAA (serotonin metabolite) was related to the improvement of OCD during treatment with clomipramine. What seems most important is that there is a decrease in the concentration of 5-HIAA and not 4-methoxy-hydroxy-phenylglycol (MHPG), the main metabolite of catecholamines, what differentiates it from depressive disorder in which there is a great decrease of the said metabolite. Flament et al. (1987) found that after a treatment with clomipramine, patients had a reduction of the activity of the monoamine oxidase by 10% and this was correlated with an improvement in the symptomatology since the activity of Platelet MAO is with the central serotonin activity.

Biological markers

Bearing in mind that the nature of the relationship (if it exists) between OCD and depression is not clear, a possible way to study it is through of the biological identification of common markers.

Dexamethasone suppression test: This test identifies an alteration in the axis hypothalamus-hypophysis-adrenal. Lieberman et al. (1985) did not find any patient with OCD that was non-suppressant, while 37% of depressed patients were not suppressors. Insel et al. (1982) found that 37% of patients with OCD, with a high score on the Hamilton scale for depression, and with a family history of depression, were non-suppressive. Vallejo et al. (1989) considered that the non-suppression that appears in patients with OCD depends on the concomitant presence of major depression.

Sleep: Patients with OCD have a shorter REM latency period, a reduction of the delta phase, a reduction of the total sleep time, and its effectiveness. There are both common aspects of both disorders when it comes to sleep.

Alterations in the central nervous system: There are differences between OCD and depressive disorder in relation to alterations in the central nervous system.

Secretion of post-clonidine growth hormone: Another biological marker of depressive disorder is the modification of the plasma concentration of the hormone growth (GH) after the administration of clonidine. This answer also appears in patients with OCD, although they do not have secondary depression (Insel et al., 1984).

Endocrine response to serotonin: The central serotonin function can be studied by measuring the concentration of hormones in the blood, whose secretion depends on hypothalamic factors that, in turn, depend on the control of serotonin. In depressive disorders, a flattened response is observed in the secretion of prolactin after stimulation with clonidine, clomipramine, or tryptophan; this alteration manifests in patients with a depressive disorder more endogenous, severe, or more melancholic. On the other hand, the results in OCD patients are quite different. One has found as high a response of prolactin secretion as in controls. From the behavioral point of view, Zohar and Colbs (1987) found that after the administration of a postsynaptic serotonin agonist (m-CPP), there produced an exacerbation of obsessive symptomatology which did not happen in the controls.

<u>OCD after the administration of placebo</u>: On the contrary, the metergoline, a blocker of serotonergic receptors, produced a decrease in its response. Depression has a flattened response in the secretion of prolactin while the OCD patients had an elevated response; both alterations can be explained through different mechanisms. In the first case, it would be due to a hyperactivity of serotonin metabolism, while the second one would be due to a down-regulation in the receivers of the serotonin.

In summary, it can be affirmed that the depressive disorder and OCD are different clinical entities, but with a high rate of comorbidity. There are depressive symptoms that appear in the course of obsessive compulsive disorder; this would correspond to a secondary depression and its response to treatment would be the same as for the rest of the symptoms of OCD. Depressive symptoms seem to correlate with some neurochemical findings. The response of OCD patients to treatment with serotonergic antidepressants is not related to the presence or absence of secondary depression.

Influence of personality in obsessive compulsive disorder

The question of the relationship between obsessive compulsive personality and OCD has long been of clinical interest and research. According to published psychoanalytic works, the two conditions are at the end of a continuum (Salzman, 1986) in which individuals with an obsessive personality differ from an obsessive neurosis in which shows egosyntonic personality traits. In this context, the obsessive compulsive personality has been considered as a factor of predisposition in the development of OCD. Janet's concept of "psychostenia" is off according to this hypothesis. However, already in the 1960s, some authors maintained that a pre-morbid obsessive personality does not represent a condition necessary or sufficient for the development of OCD (Ingram, 1961, Lewis, 1966). Various psychometric studies showed by analysis the relative independence between personality traits and obsessive symptoms (Sandíer and Hazari, 1960; Reed, 1969).

In the subsequent decade, the results of several clinical studies documented that in about one-third of patients with OCD, it is not possible to detect pre-morbid obsessive compulsive traits (Black, 1974), and that most obsessive personalities develop psychiatric conditions other than OCD (Chodoff, 1972; Morgan and Russell, 1975; Kenyon, 1976). In recent years, the debate has been revived by the DSM-III. In 1986, Rasmussen did not find a clear relationship between the personality variants described in axis II and OCD. In their work, they found a 55% association with the compulsive personality, 9% with the histrionic personality, and 7% with the schizoid.

Subsequently, several studies that used self-report instruments or interviews structured for the axis II disorder, have documented that the diagnosis of compulsive personality disorder is quite rare in patients with OCD; 0-6% while other disorders of axis II (in particular, personality disorders by avoidance, dependence, histrionics, and schizotyping) are more frequently encountered (Hoffe, 1988; Black, 1989; Baer et al., 1990; Mavissakalian et al., 1990). These results have considerable practical implications. The presence or not of obsessive compulsive personality disorder, or other disorders of axis II, could lead to different presentations of OCD or influence the response to pharmacological therapies and behavior (Jenike et al., 1986; Minichiello et al., 1987). Cassano et al. (1994) assessed the prevalence of individual personality disorders in a sample of patients (thirteen men and eighteen women) who met the criteria DSM-III diagnostics for OCD, and of a control group matched by age and sex. The results indicated that personality disorders are very frequent in patients with OCD, and those diagnosed most frequently belong to group C: in particular, avoidance (32.2%), passive-aggressive (29%), and compulsive (19.3%).

Regarding compulsive personality disorder, the prevalence shown in the group (19.3%) is certainly lower than that shown in clinical studies carried out before of the introduction of the DSM-III (Black, 1974), although consistent with the combination. Most research based on the DSM-III (Frost et al., 1994) found that personalities who are more perfectionists and with more feelings of guilt are those that are also associated with more frequency to OCD. They also found that parents were more overprotective, perfectionists, and with high levels of criticism. However, these authors considered that the definition of compulsive personality disorder as given in the DSM-III is excessively restrictive and is applicable only to the most serious and incapacitating cases

(Goldstein, 1985). The changes in the DSM-III-r have approximated the definition of the disorder in question to the traditional concept of obsessive personality (Goldstein, 1985). This is likely to generate a higher prevalence of this disorder in patients with OCD (Raer et al., 1990). On the other hand, clinical studies made prior to the introduction of the DSM-III were essentially based on a retrospective evaluation, while current research assesses co-morbidity between OCD disorders of axis II. Pollack (1987) stressed that studies based on a hindsight evaluation may favor the discovery of a much closer relationship between personality traits and OCD. It is possible that the severity of the obsessive symptoms, especially in patients with a long history of the disease, is an important factor of error in the assessment of disorders of axis II. This problem has already been recognized for other psychiatric syndromes, especially depressive and anxious syndromes (Reich et al., 1986; Mavissakalian et al., 1990).

Social interactions in obsessive compulsive disorders

Santayana (1905-1906) described the human being as a being capable of resisting his impulses and "for not letting go". According to this, psychiatric disorders can be divided into those characterized by excessive impulsivity and others characterized by excessive control. Disorders in which the fundamental problem is a lack of adaptation would be classified separately. English literature began to speak of, 'moral madness.' The impulsive madness term was widely used in German literature, and Jaspers (1909) published a paper on this, referring to the "morriña" (homesickness). At the end of the 1960s, the impulsivity began to be considered as an important part of suicidal tendencies in adolescents (Montgomery and Montgomery 1982a and 1982b). OCD has always been characterized by an extreme degree of impulse control, yet it is not surprising that in English literature, the resistance has been considered as the main psychopathological characteristic of these patients.

The conflict between social norms and individual principles has been involved in the development of mental disorders. Durkheim (1897) introduced the concept of "anomie" to describe a particular form of suicide in those individuals who thought their own principles and values were not relevant, and that they lost connection with the community; though the opposite can also happen. Kraus (1977) described the premorbid characteristics of the depressive personality from a social perspective; Tellenbach (1983) described the pre-depressive personality (melancholic type). Depressed patients show a way to adapt to social norms that Lopez-Ibor (1991) called dysnomy. So patients with obsessions and compulsions to cleaning are always dirty because they are afraid of pollution, and their compulsions are based on a control rather than on an efficient cleaning behavior. In the same way, those who have obsessions related to moral issues are those that present a more immoral lifestyle since their principles are selfish and they forget about other people. Another important aspect of OCD which is often described in the psychoanalytic literature is the aggressiveness directed against oneself. Aggression is essential for survival, but in OCD, it becomes a form of self-destructive behavior. This aspect was called by Freud as "the death instinct" or "thanatos."

The first descriptions of OCD contain very rich information about the social interaction of this disorder. Legrand du Saulle described the "folie du doute" in 1875 as a form of the four characteristics of the conscience. He distinguished three stages in the evolution of this disorder:

1) Unconfessed obsessions.
2) Obsessions that are communicated because there is a need to reaffirm.
3) Social influence.

Janet (1903) considered three stages in the evolution of OCD that could be normalized during the treatment:

1) Psychogenic stage
2) Forced agitations.

3) Obsessions and compulsions.

The psychasthenic state is equivalent to the obsessive personality- the patient feels that everything he does is imperfect; "Mental insufficiencies" are also present, some of which are volitional (indecision, procrastination, tardiness, difficulty in completing tasks that have been started), difficulty in starting new tasks and other mental insufficiencies or somatic (attention, concentration, memory). The main problem in this is control of their mental activity (thought, response to events) and their social behavior (inability to complete tasks). All this shows that the social interactions of this disorder already appear in very early stages. Hoehn-Saric and Cols (1981) described children with obsessive compulsive disorders as "poor to control their impulses." The state of forced agitation is characterized by a need for perfection, order, and symmetry. Gebstattel (1954) and López Ibor (1950-1966) described it as an important aspect of the symptomatology of OCD; the fear to finish what is being done. In the third state is when the resistance appears. Patients cannot take decisions because contrary tendencies that oppose the action arise. The conflict is secondary, consequent to the volitional alterations, and not primary as defends the psychoanalytic literature. In people affected by obsessive compulsive disorder, the fundamental conflict seems to be of an effective nature- love or hate? The difficulty in making decisions would lead to behavioral inhibition, to the loss of the internal feeling of autonomy, and to the compulsive need to verify. Recent studies that allow us to visualize the functioning cerebral through PET scan or the SPECT have involved the head of the caudate nucleus and the limbic portion of the cerebral cortex orbitofrontal. In both structures, there is an increase in consumption of glucose. The brain's computer processes depend on the energy derived from glucose metabolism; this evidence is not specific to the symptom of "doubt" but if it seems to be OCD.

In the model of Thomson, Baxter, and Schwartz, the caudate nucleus has been linked to the processing of sensory information to prepare appropriate behavior. Your dysfunction allows doubts in the interpretation of sensory information to flood consciousness. Superstitious thinking and compulsive rituals would reflect the conscious attempt of the orbitofrontal cortex to attenuate the variety of these doubts that normally do not would emerge. Gomez Mont (1993) published work in which he summarized the computational model of the neocortex developed by Mumford (in which each area of the cerebral cortex would be connected to the thalamus and geometrically would be as if the thalamus freezes a seventh layer of the cortex), as well as positron emission tomography in patients with OCD. It raises the need for studies regarding specific symptoms such as doubt, apathy, or delusions (using brain imaging techniques) to better understand the neurobiological correlation of social behavior.

7 HYPOTHESIS

The Serotonin Hypothesis

From the study conducted, it can be noted that the serotonin (5-HT) hypothesis has its basis in the pharmacology of OCD. In the late 1960s, it was observed that clomipramine, the only tricyclic antidepressant with potent 5-HT reuptake blocking properties, had antiobsessional activity. Subsequently, several studies have shown that clomipramine and several other selective serotonin reuptake inhibitors (SSRIs) are effective antiobsessional agents. In fact, results were taken as evidence that serotonin plays a fundamental role in the pathogenesis of OCD. These observations have led to the examination of the serotonin system and its function in OCD patients. Peripheral markers for the 5-HT system and a number of parameters of the 5-HT function have been investigated.

These include CSF 5-hydroxyindoleacetic acid (the major metabolite of serotonin), whole blood levels of 5-HT, platelet 5-HT concentrations, and platelet imipramine binding (thought to be reflective of 5-HT uptake). The results of these studies, although not definitive, suggest that a 5-HT dysfunction is present in OCD. More detailed information has come from pharmacologic challenge studies in which compounds were administered that, acting presynaptically or postsynaptically, stimulate 5-HT transmission. In these studies, behavioral and neuroendocrine responses in OCD patients were assessed after challenges with meta-chloro-phenyl-piperazine (mCPP), intravenous clomipramine, the 5-HT precursor tryptophan, the 5-HT releasing agent fenfluramine, ipsapirone, buspirone, and sumatriptan. These studies have also yielded conflicting results, similar to those derived from the challenge studies employing the 5-HT antagonist metergoline and tryptophan depletion. Overall, about 50% of OCD patients challenged acutely with proserotonergic compounds experienced a transient worsening of obsessive symptoms. These results suggest that for some OCD patients, there would be a basal hyperactivity of the 5-HT neurotransmission system, owing either to a hypersensitivity of the postsynaptic receptors or to a hypoactivity of the presynaptic ones, which usually provide self-regulation. This could explain both the worsening of OCD symptoms after acute 5-HT stimulation and the clinical efficacy (i.e., improvement of OCD symptoms) after chronic administration of proserotonergic compounds.

The chronic administration of clomipramine or SSRIs induces an enhanced 5-HT release in the orbitofrontal cortex, probably because of the desensitization of the terminal 5-HT autoreceptors, and this has been hypothesized to be the neurobiological substratum for the effects of SSRIs in the treatment of OCD. The involvement of the presynaptic desensitization as a key step for the neurobiological mechanism of the antiobsessional response to proserotonergic compounds is also suggested by both the long latency of clinical efficacy (6 to 8 weeks, longer than the latency for the antidepressant response induced by the same compounds), and the high doses required.

Nevertheless, the fact that not all OCD patients respond to clomipramine or SSRIs, and approximately 40% of them have no clinical improvement, may reflect the biological heterogeneity of OCD phenotype already suggested by the variability of the response to acute 5-HT challenges. Thus, consideration of more homogeneous subgroups of OCD patients defined by response to biological challenges or different symptom subtypes could lead to clarification of the pathogenesis of the disease and the role of alternative hypotheses to the serotonergic one.

The Dopamine Hypothesis

There is now considerable evidence that some forms of OCD are etiologically related to GTS (57). GTS appears to be predominantly dopaminergically mediated, as evidenced by the well-documented clinical response to haloperidol and other dopamine antagonists, by the exacerbation with L-dopa and central nervous system stimulants (such as amphetamines) (59,60), and reports of lower CSF levels of the dopamine metabolite homovanillic acid (HVA) (61). Moreover, OCD patients with comorbid tic disorder or GTS are usually resistant to conventional pharmacotherapy with proserotonergic compounds and may benefit from adjuvant treatment with dopamine (DA) or DA/5-HT blockers. This body of evidence suggests that there is an involvement of DA in at least some OCD patients.

With respect to the peripheral markers of the DA transmission, normal CSF levels of HVA have been reported, whereas the administration of fenfluramine produced increased inhibition of HVA secretion. The DA involvement has been assessed by measures of growth hormone response to apomorphine, and challenge with d-amphetamine and methylphenidate, with conflicting results. The serotonin and dopamine systems interact extensively, particularly in the basal ganglia, an area that has been implicated in the pathogenesis of obsessive compulsive phenomenology by several studies. Indirect support for the involvement of both transmitter systems includes the observation of the emergence of new OCD symptoms in patients on clozapine or risperidone, atypical antipsychotics with both D2 and 5-HT2 blocking properties, together with the demonstrated antidopaminergic activity of two antiobsessional agents, clomipramine, and fluoxetine.

8 CONCLUSION AND RECOMMENDATIONS

The identification and characterization of genes important in the expression of OCD will be a major step forward in understanding the genetic and biological risk factors attributed to the expression of this disorder. In addition, this work will allow the potential identification of other nongenetic factors associated with the manifestation or amelioration of the symptoms of the disorder. On the one hand, the identification of a linked marker will permit the design of much more incisive studies to illuminate the physiologic/ biochemical etiology of OCD by examination of the gene product and its impact on the development of the disorders. On the other hand, by controlling genetic factors through the genetic case-control research paradigm, it will be possible to document more carefully the environmental and non-genetic factors important for the expression of OCD and other possibly related conditions. Studying genetic marker data together with data characterizing phenotypic expression in the context of specific environments should allow a complete examination of the contribution of genetic and non-genetic factors.

Ways through which serotonin levels can be increased

1) Taking care of one's diet to increase serotonin:

Serotonin is not present in any food. To increase its levels, we have to resort to tryptophan. This is the amino acid from which serotonin is produced. Diets rich in tryptophan increase the levels of this substance. However, our bodies do not produce it and we need to introduce it into our diet. The supplements of this amino acid are a good compliment, but never a substitute for the diet. Foods such as soy, lean meats (turkey and chicken), tuna, salmon, pineapple, banana, artichoke, egg, chocolate, and cheese provide a dose of tryptophan needed to increase the levels of this neurotransmitter. Another way to help increase your levels is through vitamin B-6. Vitamin B-6 can influence the rate at which tryptophan converts to serotonin. Foods rich in vitamin

B-6 are potatoes, legumes, whole grains, chicken, turkey, tuna, and salmon; aka: vitamins for the brain. Adding to your diet citrus fruits which are rich in vitamin C, helps to counteract the presence of cortisol in your body who is responsible for making you feel more stress in situations that you can solve if you were calm and tranquil. Likewise, adding to each of your meals proteins of animal origin and milk, since these are rich in tryptophan (an excellent amino acid), helps in the synthesis of serotonin. It is important that you broaden your knowledge regarding the potentialities offered by food, for example, banana, spinach, and chocolate, to raise this hormone in your body.

2) Exercise to increase our serotonin

The practice of exercise is an enhancer of the levels of this neurotransmitter. Studies have shown that regular exercise can be as effective as a psychopharmacological or psychotherapeutic antidepressant treatment. It was believed that to observe the antidepressant benefits of sport, a period of several weeks was necessary. However, according to a study by the University of Texas at Austin, a period of only 40 minutes has a beneficial effect on mood. Although the mechanism by which this takes place appears to be unknown, serotonin may be involved.

3) Relax and meditate

It is just as important to move the body as to stop the mind to increase serotonin levels. Yoga or meditation are two practices that help to improve mood as well as relaxation in general.

4) The novelty helps a person to produce serotonin

Introducing novelty in our life has a positive effect on the serotoninergic system. When we start a new project, we feel more animated and in a better mood. This pleasant effect on our nervous system is produced by serotonin.

5) Laughter increases serotonin levels

The relationship of serotonin with mood is two-way. We can increase the mood by increasing this neurotransmitter, but also vice versa. The induction of moods through psychotherapy is very common; laughter therapy is perhaps the best known (benefits of laughter). Another alternative is theater classes, meeting friends, watching a funny show or remembering pleasant events.

6) With the use of food supplements

Currently, there are extensive commercial options of these food supplements not only to raise serotonin but also to bring well-being to one's body.

Serotonin and the Circadian Rhythm

The differences between the physical and mental changes, according to the activities that a human being performs between day and night, are known as circadian rhythm. When a person is at rest, which is during the hours of deep sleep, the serotonin in blood levels is in its most minimum expression while during the day in daily activities, this substance reaches the optimal levels that prepare the body for proper functioning. Our organism is coupled to these hormonal rhythms and works as a two-phase system:

- The morning phase that begins with the sunrise
- The night phase that ends with sunset.

The circadian rhythm can then infer that during the morning hours, it reduces serotonin and sleep levels, increases adrenaline and norepinephrine considerably, and also keeps you in a constant state of alert, elevates cortisol levels, improves metabolism, allows non-detrimental levels of insulin in the blood, and therefore offers better mood and energy. At night, on the other hand, the level of serotonin increases producing sleep and a feeling of calmness, decreases adrenaline and alertness, reduces cortisol, metabolism, and insulin, as well as activates growth hormone and produces more fat.

Dopamine and the Dopaminergic System

The first neurotransmitter in the mammalian brain that was discovered was epinephrine (also called adrenaline). Since the body's own production of adrenaline via various

Effects of Serotonin and Dopamine in Obsessive Compulsive Disorder

intermediates - including dopamine - runs, scientists went after the discovery of the metabolic pathways first assumed, which is that the intermediates would have no further relevance in the body. Only after the discovery that the brain has a completely different distribution pattern for dopamine than for adrenaline, led scientists Arvid Carlsson, Ake Bertler, and Evald Rosengren at the Pharmacology Institute of the University of Lund (Sweden) 1958-59 to the assumption that dopamine very own importance is attached. Through this and other experiments, the researchers discovered in the corpus striatum, a central brain region, the largest dopamine concentration. Through experiments with the plant material reserpine, were they able to prove that the emptying of the dopamine stored in this brain area leads to Parkinson-like symptoms. Oleh Hornykiewicz, at the University of Vienna, was able to show a short time later by color reactions with extracts of the corpus striatum, that these brain areas in Parkinson's patients conspicuously contained little dopamine. In 1970, Ulf Svante of Euler-Chelpin and Julius Axelrod (involved in the discovery of adrenaline and norepinephrine) received the Nobel Prize in Medicine for their discoveries on the chemical transmitters in nerve endings and the mechanism of their storage, release, and inactivation. In 2000, Arvid Carlsson and other researchers won the Nobel Prize for Medicine or Physiology "for their discoveries on signal translation in the nervous system."

The DA ($C_6H_3(OH)_2$-CH_2-CH_2-NH_2) is a catecholamine produced in a wide variety of animals, both vertebrates, and invertebrates. In the majority of neurons of the central nervous system, DA acts as a precursor of noradrenaline. Only one in 106 neurons are deficient in the enzyme dopamine β-hydroxylase, and it is responsible for transforming dopamine into noradrenaline; it is in these where DA acts as a neurotransmitter (Bannon et al., 2001). The evolution of research on dopaminergic transmission dates back to the 1950s when dopamine was recognized as a neurotransmitter since its non-uniform brain distribution suggested a specific functional role, being detected for the first time in the CNS in 1958. In the 1960s, the first evidence of the link between alterations in dopaminergic transmission and some psychiatric disorders was generated. Already by the 70s, the distribution of dopamine receptors was studied and the existence of two types of dopaminergic receptors, D1 and D2, was considered (Kebabian and Calne, 1979).

Evidence supporting a dopaminergic dysfunction in OCD stems from reports of obsessive symptoms in patients with disorders related to basal ganglia such as tics/TS, Sydenhan chorea, the onset of OCD symptoms with the use of high doses of stimulants such as ecstasy (Marchesi, 2007). It is unclear in this case whether the symptoms of OCD are exacerbated by increased dopamine or by a decrease in serotonergic function. Other evidence of dopamine involvement in OCD results from studies in rats in which repeated treatment with quinpirole, a D2/D3 agonist, induced compulsive episodes. In the rat, this effect (called "the quinpirole effect") is manifested by the exaggerated preoccupation with a certain place in the environment to which the animal returns repeatedly (Dorkin, 2010).

The beneficial effects of the associated use of dopamine antagonist neuroleptics in the treatment of OCD or with comorbid tics in both children and adults, although rarely effective as primary therapy, also supports a role for dopamine dysfunction in OCD. There was also a higher density of dopamine transporters in the left caudate and putamen in the brains of OCD carriers compared to healthy controls (Van der Vee, 2004).

In the CNS, where dopamine is synthesized mainly in the substantia nigra, DA acts as a neurotransmitter activating specific receptors. In this way, the neurotransmitter intervenes in behavior, including eating behavior and cognition, motor activity, motivation and reward, sleep, mood, attention, and learning (Barry and Klawans, 1976; Wise and Rompre, 1989; Beumont et al., 1994; Szczypka et al., 1999). In the Peripheral Nervous System, dopamine is a modulator of cardiac and renal function, vascular tone, and gastrointestinal motility (Li et al., 2006). Finally, in its role as a hormone, dopamine is the main neuroendocrine regulator of prolactin secretion since the anterior pituitary gland, intervening in the regulation of the production of breast milk (Inder and Castle, 2011).

Dopamine has been a part of living organisms for nearly a billion years. Current ideas place the dopaminergic system in the expectation of something; that is, the pursuit of something intended, including the completion of an unwanted or unpleasant task, such as taking a cold shower or submitting income taxes. Dopamine is released into the neuronal synapses in a variety of circumstances from the anxiously awaited and awaited meeting, to the delivery of the income tax return, by being free from the malaise it causes. Dopamine, related to the expectation of something, is more liberated when the animal goes out looking for food, sex, or anything else intended; is also released when we are involved in a boring and unpleasant task we want or need to finish, such as finishing work on Friday afternoon.

An important role has also been proposed for dopamine; support for this includes: a) the increase in metabolisms of basal ganglia regions observed in PET scans of OCD patients; b) the appearance of OCD symptoms in disorders that affect the basal ganglia (Sydenham chorea, toxic, trauma); c) the efficacy of blocking dopaminergic agents (pimozide and haloperidol) to reinforce the effects in some OCD patients with an unsatisfactory response to SRIs; d) the evidence that fluoxetine and clomipramine exert dopaminergic and serotonergic activity.

However, it is released even when the mind represents - even without acting - what we want to achieve, that is, when we create an inner vision of what we intend. In this case, before concrete behavior, we mentally anticipate the roadmap to be followed by one or another conduct. That is why we act behind the imagined, idealized, or intended. The person who produces little dopamine has difficulty following a certain path for a long time. The current function of man's dopamine hoping to achieve something is surely an evolutionary development of other more primitive neurochemical systems that gave rise to it. Possibly similar to other archaic catecholamines such as adrenaline, which previously served as a mediator of alertness of the body and or metabolic awakening. The alert of the organism is nothing more than the clear demonstration that the animal is alive and ready to act.

The DA promotes responses not only for the initiation of positive actions but also for the negative ones; likewise, NE (norepinephrine) may increase sensitivity for both negative and positive stimuli. Otherwise, in the face of attractive activity such as finishing a course, finding the intended girlfriend, a wedding, etc., the organism increases its levels of AD and NE in neuronal synapses. Likewise, in the face of bad activities, such as studying for the college entrance examination, doing gymnastics and then taking a cold bath, etc., the organism will also increase the levels of these two neurotransmitters to enable the body's actions to anticipate the end of unpleasant behavior; that is, be happy to finish the bad job. Therefore, the production of dopamine is felt by the body as pleasant. It is not surprising to realize that its production increases when we escape from something bad, for we are glad the more distant we are from the unbearable fact.

Feelings are part of people's daily lives; perhaps all the processes of cognition and motivation are mixed or commanded by the emotional states experienced by the individual. Several studies have shown that the more pronounced production of noradrenaline and dopamine, the more it affects us positively, guides our thinking, and allows us to obtain better and greater creativity in problem-solving. At low levels of competition, challenges or requirements, increased NA (noradrenaline) tends to be pleasant, however, at high levels of demand, increased NA may cause anxiety, i.e. an exaggerated increase will produce a low conduct of efficiency and general anxiety.

The drug dopamine belongs to the group of catecholamines and is used therapeutically in shock conditions. In addition, the substance naturally occurs in the body as an important messenger in the brain (neurotransmitters). There, it conveys motivational and drive-enhancing effects. If the levels of the messenger are too low or too high, parkinsonian symptoms may occur.

Synthesis, storage, and release

The precursor of dopamine is the amino acid tyrosine which is transported to the brain and reaches the dopaminergic neurons from the extracellular space through amino acid transporters. The synthesis of the neurotransmitter takes place in the dopaminergic nerve terminals where the responsible enzymes are in high concentration, the tyrosine hydroxylase (TH), which is the limiting enzyme in the synthesis of the neurotransmitter (Nagatsu et al., 1964), and the decarboxylase of aromatic amino acids or L-DOPA decarboxylase (Cooper et al., 1996). In the dopaminergic terminals, the neurotransmitter is synthesized in the cytoplasm from where it can be released directly into the synaptic space or it can be transported to the interior of the synaptic vesicles to be released later by exocytosis (Sudhof, 1995), thanks to the influx of Ca2 + ions (Elsworth and Roth, 1997) (Figure 2).

Recaptation

In the dopaminergic terminals, there is a high-affinity transport system that plays a decisive role in the homeostasis of the neurotransmitter since it is the main neurotransmitter elimination mechanism of the synaptic space despite the presence of catabolizing enzymes (Cooper et al., 1996; Elsworth and Roth, 1997). The dopamine transporter (DAT) belongs to the family of Na+/Cl-dependent transport proteins. It consists of 12 transmembrane domains with several phosphorylation sites (Bannon et al., 2001). It is a protein membrane capable of transporting dopamine in both directions depending on the gradient, although under normal conditions, it is more common for the dopamine to be released at the synapse, then transported back to the nerve terminal and concentrated 100-1000 times (known as recapture)

(Elsworth and Roth, 1997). Both the activity and the expression of DAT have been related to a wide spectrum of psychiatric and neurological disorders including Parkinson's disease, schizophrenia, substance abuse addiction, hyperactivity and attention deficit, and eating disorders (Persico and Macciardi, 1997; Bannon et al., 2001; Greenwood et al., 2001; Gorentla and Vaughan, 2005; Levy, 2007; Kontis and Theochari, 2012).

Metabolism

Another process that helps maintain the homeostasis of DA is its biodegradation, which is carried out in two different ways. DA can undergo oxidative deamination and become 3,4-dihydroxyphenylacetic acid (DOPAC) by the action of monoamine oxidase (MAO), which has two isoforms, A and B. Subsequently, DOPAC is released outside of the terminal to be converted into homovanillic acid (HVA) by the enzyme catechol-O-methyltransferase (COMT). On the other hand, dopamine can also be converted to 3-methoxytryramine through COMT (Cooper et al.,1996; Elsworth and Roth, 1997). Despite its greater affinity for the substrate, it has a lower catalytic activity than the soluble form (Lotta et al., 1995).

The relative expression of the enzymes varies according to the cell type, brain region, and species. In humans, isoform A of MAO is found in dopaminergic and adrenergic neurons, while isoform B is located in glial cells, astrocytes, and serotonergic neurons. COMT preferably presents a postsynaptic location to dopaminergic neurons (Elsworth and Roth, 1997). However, while membranal COMT is expressed mostly in the brain (Matsumoto et al., 2003; Matsumoto et al., 2003), cytosolic COMT does so preferentially in liver, blood, and kidneys (Lotta et al., 1995).

Receptors

Once released into the synaptic space, dopamine binds to receptors located in both presynaptic and postsynaptic terminals of the dopaminergic neurons. Initially, it was proposed that there were two types of dopaminergic receptors that differed in their pharmacological and biochemical properties, which were called D1 and D2 (Kebabian and Calne, 1979). Subsequently, up to 5 receptors (D1-D5) have been cloned which have been classified into two subfamilies named according to the nomenclature of the first two identified receptors; so the D1 subfamily includes the D1 and D5 receptors, and the D2 subfamily includes the receptors D2, D3 and D4 (Dale., 2000).

The dopaminergic receptors are coupled to G protein, with one amino-terminal extracellular end, seven transmembrane domains, and one carboxyterminal intracellular end. Activation of the receptor causes the increase (receptors D1 and D5) or decrease (receptors D2, D3, and D4) of cAMP levels (Sibley et al., 1982; Andersen et al., 1990; Sunahara et al., 1990). There are dopaminergic receptors that inhibit the synthesis and release of the neurotransmitter. These autoreceptors belong to the subfamily D2 and are more sensitive to the effect of DA than postsynaptic receptors (Elsworth and Roth, 1997).

There are differences in the distribution in the CNS of the different dopaminergic receptors. With few exceptions, the receptors of the subfamily D1 predominate over those of the D2, and within the subfamily D1/D5, the D1 is the most abundant (Jaber et al., 1996). The D5 receptors are very scarce and their function is not yet clear (Strange, 2000). Within the subfamily D2/D3/D4, the D2 is predominate in the brain. The D2 receptors, like the D1 receptors, are found mainly in the places where they project the nigrostriatal and mesolimbic pathways, and to a lesser extent in the cerebral cortex and in the pituitary gland (Jaber et al., 1996; Strange, 2000).

Dopamine Action in the Central Nervous System (CNS)

Dopamine is used in the brain to communicate with the nerve cells, so it is a neurotransmitter. In certain "circuits," it communicates positive feelings ("reward effect"), which is why he - as well as serotonin - is regarded to as a happy hormone. Compared to serotonin, however, dopamine causes a longer-term increase in motivation and drive promotion. One of the diseases in which there is a lack of dopamine in the CNS is Parkinson's disease. Typical symptoms of Parkinson's include stiff muscles, trembling and a slowing down of movement up to immobility (akinesia). Since dopamine cannot cross the blood-brain barrier, it cannot be delivered directly to compensate for the brain deficiency. Instead, precursors (L-DOPA) and analogs (dopamine agonists) of the messenger are administered, which can reach the site of action in the brain. In schizophrenic or other psychotic patients, the dopamine concentration is usually elevated in certain brain areas. Here, inhibitors of the messenger substance (dopamine antagonists) are used.

Among the antipsychotics or neuroleptics, drugs such as cocaine stop the reuptake of the released messenger substance in the nerve cell (dopamine reuptake inhibitor); it comes after their consumption to an increased dopamine effect. Thus, the brain combines drug use with a reward effect, which primarily explains the addictive effects of cocaine and other drugs.

Excessive drug use often results in clinical pictures of psychosis. Dopamine can increase blood flow in certain parts of the body (such as the kidneys). It is therefore used for shock, low blood pressure, and kidney failure. However, the use is decreasing, since, for example, adrenaline or norepinephrine drugs, lower side effect potential, are available. The declining use of dopamine is explained by the relatively high side-effect potential. Injected in shock conditions, cardiac arrhythmia, headache, dyspnoea, nausea, vomiting, and either excessive blood pressure drop or excessively high blood pressure, are common (i.e. every tenth to one-hundredth patient). Dopamine is mainly used in emergency medicine. The attending physician will clarify individually whether a patient should not receive the drug for certain reasons. The effect of meal-ingested dopamine (a diet rich in fruits and vegetables such as bananas, potatoes, avocados and broccoli) is negligible because the active ingredient is rendered inactive (deactivated) shortly after ingestion.

Dopamine and Companions: Positive and Negative

Affect

Some authors consider positive and negative affect as extremes of the same continuum. Others say that during negative affect, the person has low levels of dopamine. These ideas are wrong. It can be speculated that: 1) positive affect (mood, satisfaction, alertness) is associated with increased levels of cerebral dopamine (in addition to other neurotransmitters such as noradrenaline and serotonin), although it cannot be said that cerebral dopamine causes feelings of pleasure associated with positive effect. 2) Change in cognitive processing associated with increased positive effect has been observed. 3) People with higher positive affect perceive tasks in a more pleasant, interesting, and easier way. The richness of the task is related to its complexity, variety, and diversity, and it is assumed that positive affect enables more associations for the same fact. 4) A more expressive positive effect will facilitate the probability of trying other solutions to the same problem, which can obtain a better final result.

Otherwise, positive affection, a little high (but not too much), increases the variety of searches between healthier and more pleasant alternatives, rather than among the dangerous ones; it improves performance on a variety of tasks that are indicative of creativity or innovation in problem-solving, and creates greater available memory (more souvenirs) to deal with similar situations. On the other hand, the low or flattened positive affect causes the opposite of the above reported. A person may have low positive affect (low dopamine) and high negative affect (anxiety due to stress), may have both high affections (excited and nervous), or the two lows. The very high positive affect, for example, due to the effect of some drugs, as well as some psychoses, such as Manic Bipolar Disorder, presents a very euphoric behavior (high degree of positive affection, of mood) due to a large production of dopamine. In these cases, there is an exaggeration in actions and goals at the same time, which makes the conduct little or nothing efficient, as there is no clear and continuous goal to be pursued.

However, if the release of dopamine from the cells in the ventral tegmental area correlates with positive effect, we can deduce that positive affect (enthusiasm for action) should follow the same rules; that is, it will be greater when the reward is not likely to that which is a non-routine or unexpected gain. There is evidence in the scientific literature for this: the production and elevation of positive affect involve events unlikely to occur, such as receiving an unexpected gift, winning in the Senate, succeeding in an uncertain event, achieving a difficult achievement, etc. Joy doesn't last. After the perception of enthusiasm and euphoria, the body produces a brake on the production of positive affect neurotransmitters. This will prevent the body from continuing to enjoy the initial pleasure indefinitely. The body itself produces these substances/brakes, that is, the antagonists of the released substances. These have the function of inhibiting the pleasure obtained. There is, in these cases, a decrease in actions already underway aiming at the initial goal and decrease in the pleasure obtained by the target (food, sex, conversation) consumed.

It is not difficult to remember situations that show what is described above. A tasty food becomes, after some time, indigestible; an appetizing water is inedible after a few goals, etc. After a certain time of consumption, the things we desire fervently (water, sex, sport, chat, etc.), as well as a sense of pleasure, is interrupted and we begin to have more desire to escape from the previously desired. We all realize that a highly coveted relationship causes great pleasure and emotions at its onset (greater release of dopamine). However, little by little, it is getting comfortable and "bland" (lower production of dopamine). Some believe that a very intense initial love, an overwhelming passion is associated with a high production of dopamine at the onset, in addition to a low release of serotonin, causing the individual to become impulsive and obsessive (obsessively thinking about the loved one or car). However, soon after the first meetings (or the first few days on the beautiful site, beach, office), by increasing serotonin, the passion diminishes and often ends.

Effects of Serotonin and Dopamine in Obsessive Compulsive Disorder

There are studies showing that the obese could have, genetically, disorders in some of the neurotransmitters and or the receptors, similar to the one explained previously. It is suspected that in these cases there would be little or no production of the pleasure antagonists; that is, there would be an absence of brake production; the obese would continue the pleasure of eating a lot. A second hypothesis about the obese is that although the antagonists are produced and released in normal amounts, they would have little or no action because of a defect in the receptors, that is, they would not respond to the braking orders. The receptor is where the released neurotransmitter will act, or rather, interact. The chemical substance of the neurotransmitter interacts with the substance of the receptor, giving rise to the latter, to stimuli or inhibitions. A similar fact seems to occur with some alcoholics; they just feel the well-being of the drink.

Of all sense organs, smell seems to be what most directly and immediately produces an effective response. Studies have shown that pleasant odors do not necessarily induce positive effects. On the other hand, pleasant odors help conduct and improve performance in varied tasks, just as other strategies produce positive effects, such as listening to some melody or poetry, watching a beautiful dance, playing a game, and receiving a present, preferably not expected. Unpleasant odor and pain can produce the "angry" emotion, so it is common to swearing an ugly name after hitting your knee on the table or cutting your finger when peeling an orange and becoming more aggressive in a smelly environment.

Another aspect concerns the duration that dopamine is released. Dopamine in cells (dopaminergic projection of cells in the ventral tegmental (mesolimbic) area) is released only for a few seconds before a reward. However, the elevation of positive effect caused by the present remains for 30 minutes or more. The explanations speak that the stimulation of one brain area for 10 seconds increases the release of dopamine in the acupunctural core area by more than 30 minutes. Thus, dopamine continues to be released upon cessation of stimulation. In the event that the dopaminergic system is damaged, the animal will exhibit, as a result, an inertia behavior. On the other hand, if the intact system is stimulated, electrically or pharmacologically, various actions and physiological changes are reinvigorated. We can affirm that the excitation of these circuits alters the usual sensitivity of the sensory systems, important and essential for order and coherence in the behaviors, provoked or aroused.

The electrically induced excitation of the dopaminergic system leads to more effective cortical processing related to the aroused areas, such as feeding, sex, companionship, danger, etc. Actually, the reverse is true. Decrease, such as that in Attention Deficit Disorder, leads the wearer to a constant shifting of attention by not being able to fix it on the intended or initiated goal. There also seems to be less capacity to set several possible goals at the same time. Negative (NA) or unpleasant effect is not simply the opposite of positive affect (PA) in conduct or cognition; it seems to be mediated by systems other than those related to positive effect. The decrease in dopamine is related to anhedonia (with the lowest intensity of emotion or positive effect), that is, with a flattened affection, with the loss of pleasure, and without will (abulico), with depression. The depressed person, even slightly, has his ability diminished in solving difficulties because he thinks slowly, has his mental representations poorer, and a more negative imagination. Antidepressants, when they produce results, transform the way of "seeing and deciphering the world" of the depressed. However, this hypothesis about catecholaminergic depression is limited and incomplete.

In negative affection, there are diverse emotions or affections, all of them unpleasant, usually associated with the stressful events faced such as anxiety (fear), phobia, anger, among others. It is not uncommon to experience such indifference, laziness, and poor productivity in individuals using antihypertensive drugs, anti-histamines, and anti-anxiety medications. Finally, these drugs are drugs that have the opposite effect of cocaine and amphetamine; that is, they do not cause euphoria and well-being, but rather discomfort and discouragement. This picture of apathy is caused by the

Effects of Serotonin and Dopamine in Obsessive Compulsive Disorder

depletion (docking of the neurotransmitter) of dopamine in the acupuncture nucleus. Among these psychiatric drugs are those used in the treatment of patients with schizophrenia, mania, and other disorders: Haldol or Haloperidol, Amplictil, Stelazine and several others.

These drugs, in addition to blocking the effects of dopamine (antagonists), also produce bizarre effects, such as those of dysfunctional movements, increase the difficulty of learning and remembering, and often make these patients less motivated. In all these cases, there is often a decrease in positive affect and, therefore, discouragement, fatigue, less physical and cognitive capacity; these signs and symptoms vary with the person and the dosage. This condition improves by decreasing or stopping the medication, and by the use of some substances, among them biperiden, also used for the treatment of Parkinson's disease. This medicine is intended to increase the release of dopamine.

Emotional circuits can be stimulated by perceptions of

things, events or events in the environment that are conditioned (linked) or associated with pleasure or suffering at the instant of fact. The dopaminergic mesolimbic system exhibits a vigorous release of dopamine during the anticipatory phase of appetitive-conditioned behavior; that is before the individual achieves the desired goal, such as succulent steak. In this case, various environmental factors which were previously neutral become "linked" to the pleasures or sufferings that have arisen. In the case of steak, the person can remember it in front of a similar smell, when passing the restaurant where he ate the steak, when talking about delicious food, etc. We all have our joyful, sad, or enthusiastic memories as we listen to certain melodies that have been heard during our periods of happiness or suffering.

Dopamine - Memory, Hippocampus, and Acetylcholine

The hippocampus is a temporal lobe structure that is necessary for the consolidation of episodic memory (memory of episodes as the first day of school, etc.). The normal function of the hippocampus (of this sector of memory) depends critically on the neurotransmitters acetylcholine and dopamine. Studies show that the decline of these neurotransmitters (due to use of antipsychotic medications, Parkinson's disease, Alzheimer's) produces memory problems. It appears that dopamine - released during increased positive effect - in turn, leads to an increased release of acetylcholine in the hippocampus. It seems that the neutral material that is stored in the memory is organized around positive or negative effect, especially in extreme cases. We remember the facts because of the emotions they provoked. However, under normal circumstances, most people use positive affects rather than negatives to organize and store memory. While many people seem to enjoy the so-called negative emotions, such as those triggered by the sight of horror, adventure and action movies, watching TV, newspapers, or even live catastrophes, all of these can awaken people. In movies, there is almost always the provocation of anxiety, fear, horror, anger, sadness, and even disgust. It is possible that these states release more dopamine. If these studies are correct, a new hypothesis of improving our memory opens: is it enough to increase our sources of pleasure and to diminish our negative emotions?

Inhibitors of Serotonin Reuptake/Serotonin Antagonists: Trazodone

Trazodone is an antidepressant that acts by blocking serotonergic 5-HT2A receptors with a secondary serotonin reuptake inhibition action. It also possesses antihistamines and α1-antagonist actions. Given its serotonergic action, trazodone has been tested on its own in the treatment of OCD. The first case report dates back to 1984, which reported the case of a patient treated with trazodone, 100 mg/day, who experienced a significant improvement in obsessive, compulsive and depressive symptoms after 4 weeks of treatment. The same observation was reported by Baxter the following year on two patients with OCD. Ramchandani described a further case of trazodone treatment of a patient with bowel obsession (obsessive fear of public display of borborygmi or losing control of the sphincters): patient responded to treatment with 150 mg/day of trazodone in just 3 weeks, complete remission of symptoms was present at a follow-up visit after 18 months.

There is an observational study of 8 obsessive compulsive patients in monotherapy with trazodone: 6 obtained a significant improvement of obsessive compulsive symptomatology after 4 weeks, a detectable improvement even at a follow-up of 6 weeks. A similar observation was reported on a sample of 9 patients with OCD resistant to treatment with clomipramine. The sample showed a slight but significant improvement in treatment with trazodone, reporting relapse to therapy discontinuation and responding again to its reacquisition. Based on these preliminary observations, a double-blinded, placebo-controlled study was performed on a sample of 21 patients with OCD. Patients were treated for 10 weeks with trazodone (average dose 235 mg/day) or placebo. The two groups of patients did not differ from each other due to the severity of obsessive, compulsive and depressive symptoms. At the end of the observation, there were no significant differences between patients treated with trazodone and patients treated with placebo.

Selective Inhibitors of Serotonin and Norepinephrine Re-Uptake: Venlafaxine

Venlafaxine is a serotonin and norepinephrine reuptake inhibitor, its mechanism of action is similar to that of tricyclics, but is not burdened by the anticholinergic, antihistamine and α-blocker effects of the latter. Regarding its use in the treatment of OCD, there are some case reports of patients resistant to SSRIs or intolerant to their side effects. Zajecka et al. described the case of a refractory patient to other drugs treated with venlafaxine, 375 mg/day who responded within 5 weeks; however, the response criteria used to evaluate the efficacy of venlafaxine were not specified. Ananth et al. reported the case of two patients - resistant or intolerant to SSRIs - treated with venlafaxine (150 mg/day) successfully.

Grossman & Hollander, who treated a patient intolerant to clomipramine and paroxetine with venlafaxine monotherapy, 225 mg/day, described another case report. After 5 weeks of treatment, the patient's Y-BOCS score (Yale-Brown Obsessive Compulsive Scale) dropped from 24 to 7 and the patient continued to show a positive response even after 10 months. In the same year, another study was carried out on a sample of 10 patients (all subjects never treated with a drug therapy or subjects resistant to previous treatments with SSRI) who were treated with venlafaxine doses between 150 and 375 mg/day (mean dose = 308 mg/day).

Responsive patients showed a reduction in the Y-BOCS score ≥35% of the initial value and a score at the CGI (Clinical Global Impressions) ≥ 2 at the end of the 12 weeks of treatment. In accordance with these criteria, venlafaxine was effective in 3 patients (30%). Interestingly, these 3 patients were all unprecedented psychopharmacological treatments, while the 7 non-venlafaxine patients had an average of 2.5 previous failed treatments. A single-blinded study conducted over a period of 12 weeks compared the efficacy of venlafaxine with that of clomipramine in the treatment of OCD on a sample of 65 patients. The response was evaluated at Y-BOCS and CGI-I, using the same criteria reported by the aforementioned study of Rauch et al. In both groups, there was a significant reduction of obsessive-compulsive symptoms, with no significant difference between patients treated with clomipramine and those treated with venlafaxine.

In fact, patients treated with venlafaxine reported better tolerability to the drug. In another open-label study, 39 patients with OCD, of whom 29 were resistant to first choice therapies, were treated with venlafaxine up to 230 mg/day doses. Of these, 27 (69.2%) were considered responders with a CGI-I score of 2 (much improved) or 1 (very much improved). The mean final score at CGI-I of the whole sample was 1.9 ± 1.06. There is only one double-blinded, randomized, placebo-controlled study of the use of venlafaxine in OCD. It was conducted over a period of 8 weeks using a sample of 30 patients treated with 225 mg/day of venlafaxine or placebo;

the response to therapy was evaluated with CGI-I. At the end of the study, there were no significant differences between venlafaxine and placebo; there was, however, a trend of significance in favor of a better response to venlafaxine in the 8-week period. The authors concluded that patients treated with venlafaxine would probably have received greater benefit from the drug over a longer period of time than in the study and with doses higher than 225 mg/day.

No other controlled studies with placebo were performed to confirm the efficacy of venlafaxine in OCD. However, in 2003 Denys et al. conducted a comparative, randomized, double-blinded study with paroxetine, on a total sample of 150 patients. Both in patients treated with venlafaxine (300 mg/day) and in patients treated with paroxetine (60 mg/day), the Y-BOCS score is reduced by about 40% from the initial condition. There were no significant differences between the two groups as regards the proportion of patients responsible for treatment: in the venlafaxine group 28 patients (37%) were partially responsive, 18 patients

(24%) were responsive to the drug; in the paroxetine group 33 patients (44%) were partially responsive, 17 patients (22%) were responsive to the drug. In a second study conducted by the same authors on the same sample 36, after a period of pharmacological washout, 16 patients resistant to paroxetine were treated with venlafaxine and 27 patients resistant to venlafaxine were shifted to paroxetine. At the end of the study, the percentage of patients responsive to treatment was 56% for paroxetine and 19% for venlafaxine. These data suggest a lower efficacy of venlafaxine in the treatment of patients with non-responsive SSRIs.

Specific Noradrenergic and Serotonergic Antidepressants: Mirtazapine

The main pharmacological action of mirtazapine is antagonism on α2-adrenergic receptors. It also blocks three serotonergic receptors: 5-HT2A, 5-HT2C, and 5-HT3, in addition to histamine H1 receptors (Fig. 1). When α2-presynaptic heteroceptors are blocked, the presynaptic release of serotonin increases, the action of which occurs on 5-HT1A receptors, because the other serotonergic receptors are blocked by the drug. Mirtazapine was tested as monotherapy for OCD in the first open-label study (at a dose of between 15 and 45 mg/day) in 10 patients. The mean decrease in symptomatology measured at Y-BOCS was 2.7 ± 6.3 points; there were two patients that responded to the therapy.

The authors concluded that mirtazapine did not seem to be a valid treatment for OCD, although definitive conclusions required a study conducted on a larger sample. The same authors retested the drug in a subsequent study conducted on 30 subjects with OCD treated with mirtazapine from 30 mg/day up to 60 mg/day for 12 weeks. At the end of the study, 16 patients (53.3%) were considered responders. There was no difference in the response rate even when the patients were divided into drug-naive patients and patients who had shown resistance to previous treatments. The most important side effects observed were asthenia and weight gain. In a second phase of the study, subjects responded to a double-blinded, randomization to receive placebo or to continue therapy with mirtazapine for another 8 weeks. The patients who continued the mirtazapine therapy fell in a lower percentage compared to those treated with placebo (29% vs. 62%), however, the difference was not statistically significant.

Inhibitors of Dopamine and Norepinephrine Reuptake: Bupropion

Bupropion is a dopamine and norepinephrine reuptake inhibitor, effective in the treatment of depression and social phobia. In Italy, this drug is indicated only as an adjuvant for smoking cessation. Vulink et al. have recently carried out an open-label study on 12 patients to investigate the efficacy of monotherapy bupropion in the treatment of OCD (a possible involvement of the dopaminergic system in OCD is in fact suggested by the efficacy of the use of low-dose antipsychotics as an add-on of serotonergic therapy in cases of resistant OCD). The study lasted 8 weeks, using a maximum drug dose of 300 mg/day. The mean decrease in the Y-BOCS score of the whole sample was 1.1 ± 9.6 and is not significant. Only two patients could be considered responsive to treatment, with an average decrease to Y-BOCS of 31%.

Benzodiazepines: Alprazolam, Clonazepam

Benzodiazepines are drugs that bind to a receptor component for γ-aminobutyric acid (GABA) type A, located on the neuronal membranes of the central nervous system. These are easy-to-agonist; the action of GABA acting as positive allosteric modulators of the receptor function. There are some case reports in the literature regarding the use of alprazolam in OCD. The first case report concerning the use of this drug in OCD treatment dates back to 1984 due to the anxiety that accompanied his obsessions and panic attacks; a man suffering from OCD had been treated with alprazolam with a clear reduction of obsessions and disappearance of compulsions. A similar case was reported two years later. In an observation on a small sample of 4 patients, all diagnosed with OCD according to the DSM-III-r criteria and treated with alprazolam on monotherapy, showed an improvement of obsessive symptoms, anxiety, and with consequent improvements in mood tone.

More data is available for clonazepam, a 7-nitro-benzodiazepine with some effects also on the serotoninergic system. Several case reports and open-label studies have suggested that clonazepam has anti-obsessive properties. Bodkin & White treated a 21-year-old OCD patient with clonazepam that, at 1 mg/day, led to complete remission of the compulsions and at 3 mg/day resulted in the complete disappearance of obsessions and anxiety. Bacher observed the efficacy of clonazepam in the treatment of a 60-year-old man with OCD, resistant to treatment with other benzodiazepines. Hewlett et al. described the case of 3 patients with OCD who responded successfully to treatment with clonazepam and Ross & Pigott reported the case of a 14-year-old teenager who showed a reduction in obsessive thoughts after treatment with monotherapy with clonazepam at 2 mg/day.

Effects of Serotonin and Dopamine in Obsessive Compulsive Disorder

In a double-blinded study, 28 subjects with OCD diagnosis according to DSM-III-r criteria were randomized into 4 samples treated for 6 weeks afterward with clomipramine, clonazepam, clonidine, and diphenhydramine (a drug without any efficacy on OCD). Clomipramine and clonazepam were both more effective than the control drug in reducing obsessive compulsive symptoms. Forty-percent of patients not responsive to clomipramine only achieved clinically significant improvement through clonazepam treatment. The improvements induced by clonazepam were not related to the decrease in anxiety and occurred in the first days of treatment. Clonazepam was significantly more effective than the other three drugs during the first 3 weeks of treatment. Based on these preliminary data, Hollander et al. implemented a randomized, double-blinded, placebo-controlled study of a sample of 27 patients with OCD. Regarding the decrease in the obsessive symptomatology, from the measurements to Y-BOCS and CGI-I, there was no significant difference in the response to the drug between the two groups. Two patients treated with placebo were found to be responsible, only one among those treated with clonazepam responded to therapy.

Neuroanatomic Substrate

Another contribution of the Rapoport theory on OCD was to direct the research on the neuroanatomic substrate of OCD to the nuclei of the base. This is because the striatum is a critical structure for the organization of innate behaviors, such as self-cleaning routines and territorial boundaries. In fact, functional neuroimaging techniques of the brain point to dysfunction of the caudate nucleus, added to the orbitofrontal cortex, and to the thalamus in OCD. Particularly relevant to the present analysis are the works by Baxter et al in California. Using scanning with positron emission tomography (PET scan), these researchers described a hyperactivation of the three structures listed above in patients with OCD. This finding is suggestive that a reverberation of the caudate-thalamus-frontal circuit is responsible for obsessive compulsive manifestations. Supporting this hypothesis, results obtained in the same laboratory showed that the two most effective therapeutic procedures - SSRI medication, in this case, fluoxetine, and cognitive-behavioral therapy - eliminated the aforementioned hyperactivation identified by PET. Not forgetting that the greater impact of these findings were to document, for the first time, a neurophysiological alteration determined by a modality of psychotherapy, the fact that a modular SSRI of striatal activity again refers to 5-HT and gives a valuable clue as to which serotonergic system and type most likely to be involved in OCD.

Mesostriatal serotonergic system and 5-HT receptors

It is known that the serotonergic innervation of the forebrain comes from two nuclei located in the midbrain: the median raphe nucleus and the dorsal raphe nucleus. While fibers originating in the median raphe nucleus are mainly projected in limbic structures, those originating in the dorsal raphe nucleus predominantly innervate the nuclei of the base and the neocortex. In view of the anatomical and functional evidence discussed above, it can be deduced that the serotonergic pathway from the dorsal raphe nucleus and projected in the caudate is the most likely candidate to participate in the pathophysiology of OCD.

As for 5-HT receptors, it is known that they are subdivided into several types and subtypes whose cellular and anatomical location, as well as the functional role, are equally different. Of particular note is the fact that receptors of the 5-HT 1B/1D subtype are selectively concentrated in the striatum. The double denomination 1B/1D comes from the diversity in pharmacological profile. For example, propranolol blocks the 5-HT 1B receptor, but not 5-HT 1D. The former occurs in certain species, such as the rat, and the second, in others, including humans. Moreover, they resemble everything, particularly with regard to location and function. These are presynaptic receptors, located on the membrane of the varicosities of terminal nerve fibers, from which 5-HT is released by the action of the nerve impulse. Stimulation of 5-

HT 1B/1D receptors decreases the amount of 5-HT thus released. Therefore, such receptors have a regulatory role on the release of the neurotransmitter, limiting it when the amine concentrations in the synaptic cleft reach high levels. It is, therefore, the well-known mechanism of negative feedback.

Hypothesis on the Role of 5-HT in OCD

In addition to the anatomical disposition, the idea that 5-HT 1D receptors participate in the pathophysiology of OCD has gained important pharmacological support with the finding that the selective 5-HT 1D agonist sumatriptan aggravates the symptoms of patients with OCD. This evidence adds up to previous results with the less selective agent meta-chlorophenylpiperazine (mCPP). In this case, it was also found that chronic treatment with clomipramine abolished the aggravating effect of mCPP. As SSRIs reduce the sensitivity of the 5-HT1B/1D receptor to agonists after prolonged use, it was hypothesized that receptor subtype would be supersensible in OCD. As a result, there would be less release of 5-HT in the mesothelial serotonergic pathway, with reduction of 5-HT synaptic concentration in the striatum, resulting in activation of the caudate-thalamic-frontal circuit responsible for the manifestations of OCD. Indeed, a single-photon emission computed tomography (Spect) study showed increased hyperactivity of these structures during symptomatic aggravation induced by sumatriptan. It can be concluded that there is suggestive evidence that the supersensitivity of 5-HT 1D presynaptic receptors, located in the mesothelial serotonergic pathway, is responsible for the disinhibition of the caudate-thalamic-cortical circuit, which generates the compulsive symptoms of OCD. The chronic administration of SSRIs would decrease the sensitivity of the same receptors, improving the clinical picture.

OCD and Streptococcal infections

It is now known that some children develop obsessive compulsive symptoms after a streptococcal infection. Estimates are that this can be an important mechanism in 10%

to 20% of children who develop OCD. Typically, the symptoms are accompanied by tics and this phenomenon may be related to OCD symptoms seen in Sydenham chorea. It is proposed that this represents an autoimmune disorder caused by the reaction of the bacteria and the basal ganglia; several lines of research support this hypothesis. The data examined suggest that the increase in the volume of the basal ganglia is associated with the PANDAS, as well as that they are involved in OCD, disorders with tics, and Sydenham chorea. It is very common that children with disorders with tics (and perhaps OCD) present an abrupt onset and exacerbations of the infection. It has been reported that more than 50% of children with tics had this finding and 11% reported exacerbation of symptoms within 6 months after the streptococcal infection.

In one study, the basal ganglia of rats were drained and compared with serum from boys who had both a history of PANDAS and antineuronal antibodies or serum from healthy boys without antineuronal antibodies. It appeared that the rats of the first group showed stereotyped behaviors, while those of the second group did not. However, antineuronal antibodies were sought and found in children with La Tourette syndrome as well as in normal control subjects. Although patients with Tourette had higher mean levels, these researchers found no correlation between average antibody levels, clinical severity, types of symptoms, history (age of onset or precipitation), or evidence of streptococcal infections. In addition, there was no correlation between the severity of symptoms or the duration and measurement of the basal ganglia in a study of children diagnosed with PANDAS. In addition, it happens that the autoimmune mechanism is only relevant when the acute onset pattern is observed. When comparing a cohort of children with "normal" OCD with normal controls, children with attention deficit hyperactivity disorder, and children with tics, it was found that there was no correlation between the levels of antistreptolysin O, anti-Dnase B or volume of the basal ganglia and OCD. Although an autoimmune mechanism could predict the particularly high frequency of disease among the relatives of individuals with

PANDAS, it is interesting that one study did not show higher rates than those seen in OCD. In addition, the number of first-degree relatives with infant-onset of symptoms was the same as in current OCD studies and their families. Preliminary data support the efficacy of immunological treatments such as intravenous immunoglobulin and plasmapheresis, but it happens that these treatments are not useful for patients who have not had the infection related to the onset or exacerbation of PANDAS.

In 1990, the existence of a "basal-thalamus-cortical ganglia" circuit was proposed and it was suggested that a "lateral orbitofrontal" circuit projected to the ventromedial sectors of the caudate, the substantia nigra, and globus pallidus, should be involved in OCD. There were doubts about how these separate circuits would be. Subsequently, the SPECT findings led to the proposal of a similar "orbital-basal ganglia-thalamic" circuit. This basic model affirms that the cortico frontal and limbic structures have excitatory effects on striatal structures through glutamatergic references. These striatal structures, including the caudate, putamen, nucleus accumbens, and olfactory tubercle, project to the inner and outer part of the globus pallidus. From the inner part of the globus pallidus, inhibitory references using aminobutyric acid have tonic activity in the thalamus. Consequently, the increased striatal activity decreases the inhibitory activity (or creates disinhibition) in the thalamus. The increased activation in the thalamic nucleus produces excitatory transmission to the cortical structures and then movement.

The corticothalamocortical circuit is affected in several ways in OCD during its treatment. However, this basic model has required modifications in two ways. The first modification introduces separate direct and indirect pathways between the thalamus and the striatum. The direct route is very fast because it passed directly from the striatum to the thalamus, thus exerting a disinhibition effect (activation). On the other hand, the indirect path sends several stimuli to the subthalamic nucleus, which, in turn, sends stimuli to both the internal and external part of the globus pallidus. The indirect way moderates activity in the thalamus. The second modification proposes two parallel systems of the striate, one connected to the dorsolateral region and the other to the ventromedial region.

The entrance of the ventromedial region is largely from the limbic structures, while the dorsolateral regions receive inputs from the dorsal cortex. In OCD, the tone excessively increased in the pathway from the limbic cortex to the ventromedial striatum, activates the direct pathway, decreases inhibition, and produces symptoms (overactivation) (Baxter, 1999). The treatment with SSRIs (the afferents to the ventromedial way) is attenuated at the level of the striatum; the tone of the direct path decreases in relation to the dorsal system, and balance is restored. Baxter (1999) states that the behavioral treatment acts to increase the tone of the dorsolateral system in relation to the ventromedial system; increasing the tone in the dorsolateral system restores the balance.

Psychoanalytic Theories

Freud classified it as a psychoneurosis. He said that the cause was caused by an alteration in the sexual life or development of the child that goes through the oral, anal, and sexual interest (Oedipus stages). During or before the oral phase, there is a conflict between the ego (the organized self) and the id (the instinctive self). The ego solves the conflict by trying to reduce the effect of the id, even if the solution is not pleasant. A situation could be to return to the development phase (anal) and accumulate (not want to throw anything). Another regression, for example, to check the oven is interpreted as a way to deal with an aggressive desire to burn the house. Today this has more to do with the problems of development, which produces a disorder in the personality, but not OCD.

Freud considers that the majority of obsessive symptoms, especially those of shame and exaggerated scruple, originate in the inability to defend oneself from the unconscious, aggressive tendencies that originate during the anal phase. During this period, strongly aggressive and sexual tendencies emerge and the ego is too weak to defend itself against the prohibitions of the super-ego, as a result, the ego responds with symptoms of scrupulousness, cleanliness, and mercy, and the libidinous impulses pass from the genital organization to the anal-sadistic. As a consequence of the dysfunction of the two egos, obsessive neuroses appear. This coincides with other findings because the frontal lobe is involved in the inhibition or modification of aggressive and sexual impulses, and may be impaired in OCD. Due to the deficit of these egos, Freud proposes that patients with obsessive neuroses are not successful in their control of ambivalence, including the resolution of aggressive and sexual urgencies, or "intrasystemic contradictions" such as feelings of love-leisure, masculinity-femininity, and others. Similarly, characteristics of avoidance, intellectualization, reactive training, and isolation are very prominent in OCD.

Cognitive theories

These theories suggest that obsessions represent catastrophic misunderstandings in the thoughts, images, and impulses of an individual. Examples of flaws in the cognitive processes would be perfectionism, intolerance to insecurity, and excess of anguish to the threat.

Differential Diagnosis

A differential diagnosis depends on the classification system used to define OCD. There are many disorders in which obsessions and compulsions can be seen, such as anorexia nervosa, dysmorphobia, depression, hypochondriasis, obsessive compulsive personality disorder, organic mental disorder, panic, phobias, post-traumatic stress, schizophrenia, schizotypal personality, trichotillomania, somatization, somatoform disorder, Tourette syndrome, "fear of AIDS," disorder with illusions (all types), and generalized developmental disorder. Although rare, there are specific brain disorders (organic brain syndromes) that present OCD.

Special care must be taken not to equate subclinical obsessions-compulsions with OCD, especially in adolescents, since these phenomena appear to be stable characteristics that do not interfere with development. Inexperienced clinicians confuse obsessive compulsive personality disorder (OCPD) with OCD, when in fact most OCD patients do not develop OCPD. Although people with OC personality (OCPD) may have rigid routines, need for order, accumulation, and indecision behaviors, they usually do not experience this as egodystonic; their behaviors generally do not generate anxiety or deterioration, and the latter when it appears it is due to belief patterns and behaviors, and not the symptoms themselves. On the contrary, patients with OCD are not emotionally cold, expressionless, greedy or especially rigid in moral or ethical matters. In addition, accumulation, preparation of lists, and rigid schedules are not common among compulsions reported by patients with OCD. Recently, a group of patients with proven OCD and their relatives were systematically evaluated, comparing them with a control group, verifying that the former showed high rates of obsessive compulsive *personality* disorder. This could suggest the hypothesis of a "spectrum" of conditions that includes OCD and OCPD, and that exhibits vertical transmission.

Differentiating psychosis from overestimated ideas of obsessive patients can be cumbersome. DSM-IV establishes the possibility of coexistence of schizophrenia or disorders with illusions, with OCD. For these differentiations, it is important to consider that patients with OCD have positive self-criticism (insight) to know that their obsessions originate in their own minds and are not imposed by external forces. Clinicians should consider that it is comorbid pathology when there is no self-criticism. "Fear of AIDS," consists of obsessive fear and worries about getting AIDS. Clinicians cannot make a reliable diagnosis of hypochondriasis if one takes into account the long incubation period of the disease. Many cases are between subthreshold obsessions and OCD.

Clinical Evaluation

This is the first critical step in the treatment of OCD. A proper evaluation must include several sources. A story should be made with the patient alone, with the parents/spouses alone, and with the family gathered. Useful information can be obtained from teachers about their academic or work performance, relationships with classmates or friends, areas of deterioration, and tasks that represent special difficulties. Siblings can provide valuable information about the family's responses to the patient.

Children often feel ashamed of their symptoms and the deterioration they cause, thus often fearing that their symptoms are rare and crazy. They are very likely to describe their symptoms to clinicians who know how to resist confrontation, transmit acceptance, and respect privacy, but may take a while to fully reveal their fears, so it will not be easy to conduct a full evaluation in one session. The objectives of the individual meetings are to estimate the magnitude of the deterioration, the level of development, the symptoms that are progressing and the associated diagnoses. Clinicians need to know the patient's strengths and weaknesses, fears and aspirations, successes and failures. The deterioration produced by the symptoms generally reaches home, school, work, relationships with colleagues and self-image. This involves evaluating the patient's fit in each of these fields. Although there is a temptation to meet with the patient to try to discover things that he has denied, to unveil secrets, or unmask obsessions, fostering a relationship with the patient is critical. It is a very common mistake to enroll in an effort to eradicate the symptoms and overcome the concealment that the patient makes of them.

The family can provide information about the extent to which the symptoms interfere with the patient's life, but it can also help to perpetuate the symptoms. Situationally, genetically, and psychologically, OCD can be a family disorder. The purpose of evaluating the family is to know the prevailing family dynamics and to identify the extent to which the patient's symptoms affect the family. This involves knowing the meaning of the patient's symptoms for their parents (in the case of children), how the parents understand their child, and the family's response to the child's behaviors. These purposes will be more truly completed with direct intervention and interaction with the family. A critical question is whether a concomitant treatment of the family may be necessary to change the patterns of communication, filial relationships, and clarify reasons for conflict. When the psychopathology of the parents aggravates the patient's condition, treatment of them may be necessary.

The meeting with the parents alone serves both to educate them and to obtain information from them. Facts about the parents and their marriage, partner conflicts, concerns and frustrations about their child, and potentially confidential information about the family history or their own symptoms should be obtained without the patient. A second great purpose of the meeting with the parents alone is to teach and reassure them about their child's illness. They may fear that their child is psychotic or intractable, feel guilty that they may have provoked their child's situation, or fear that clinicians will blame him for their difficulties or compete with them for their affection. These meetings are an opportunity to reassure them and solidify a collaborative relationship with parents.

Creating a space where symptoms and pressure can be discussed and monitored may not achieve a complete review of all the fields that cause distress and difficulty. Standardized instruments can be more effective for a general evaluation and selection; although, they may not allow the symptoms and their impact to be evaluated qualitatively, they will review a series of behaviors and fields while allowing to assess the severity in comparison with a clinical population.

There are no specific laboratory studies for OCD and the clinical findings should always be used first. The electrocardiogram, hemogram, liver, and kidney function may be necessary before starting pharmacotherapy. Copper levels are unnecessary in the absence of psychotic symptoms or physical signs of tics or chorea. Only when signs of local focusing are observed, would the CT and the resonance be indicated. Karyotypes can be obtained in patients with abnormal appearance. The electroencephalogram is only indicated when a seizure disorder is suspected.

Psychological tests provide insight into the intellectual function, severity of acute stressors, and characteristics of defensive structures in patients with OCD. Standardized tests such as the Wechsler Intelligence Scale for Children (WISC-III) or the Kaufman Assessment Battery for Children (K-ABC), for younger children, are appropriate for determining the intellectual level. Projective tests like the Rorschach, Thematic Apperception Test, or draw-a-person to identify sources of stress, are very ambiguous. The multiphasic personality inventory for adolescents can be useful to identify current stressors and characteristic defense patterns. Measures of severity of obsessions and compulsions are being discussed. In addition, the child-parent version of the child behavior catalog or the behavioral assessment system for children can help discover other maladaptive behaviors.

Treatment

Obsessive compulsive disorder (OCD) can be effectively controlled in 75% of cases with an adequate treatment that usually includes the use of psychotropic drugs and psychotherapy, although in very serious cases it may be necessary to resort to other techniques, such as neurosurgery, also called psychosurgery. The finding that serotonin secretion was altered in patients with OCD opened an important route for pharmacological treatment. At present, the drugs of choice are the so-called selective serotonin reuptake inhibitors (SSRIs), which include fluoxetine, fluvoxamine, paroxetine, and sertraline. The so-called serotonin and noradrenaline reuptake inhibitors (SNRIs) have also been incorporated into the therapeutic armamentarium, including venlafaxine and mirtazapine. The latter is used when treatment fails with the previous ones or in cases in which OCD is associated with depression. Eighty-percent of patients with OCD shows some type of response to pharmacological treatment, although only in half of them there is a clear remission of symptoms and the decrease in frequency and intensity of both obsessive thoughts and compulsions. However, it should be noted that although these drugs are generally well tolerated, they must be administered at high doses and for a prolonged period; and that the improvement might take a few weeks to occur.

There is evidence that combination therapies with SSRIs and CBT in children with OCD are superior to placebo, with good tolerability, and more effective than CBT or sertraline alone, probably because of a synergistic effect. In adults, the benefits of combination therapy are less clear; CBT appears to be superior to clomipramine (and, in another study, better than SSRIs potentiated with risperidone), without significant improvement when using both strategies. Although in these studies, expert professionals carried out intensive CBT and the medication was generally administered in inflexible schemes. There are reports of polymorphisms in enzymes that metabolize some drugs used to treat OCD, associated with resistance to treatment and adverse effects. The authors conclude that the treatment of OCD is not yet adequate since many patients do not respond to it or suffer recurrences. SSRIs represent the first line of treatment for OCD since their efficacy and tolerability are high. It is suggested to use them at high doses and for a long time. Clomipramine is an adequate alternative but is associated with effects that are more adverse. When monotherapy fails, it is suggested to potentiate these drugs with neuroleptics at low doses (especially risperidone) or psychotherapy, but there are not many alternatives in case of failure of these strategies.

Varieties of treatments have been applied to children with OCD although only behavioral therapy and medications have been systematically studied. Joint family treatment and individual psychotherapy were generally also required. Hospitalization was required in some circumstances. All means will be used because the clinician's relationship with the patient is crucial for several reasons. First, most children with OCD are apprehensive and reserved; they are anxious about their symptoms and the treatment, and the relationship with the clinician can reassure and diminish much of their anxiety, preferably in a way that promotes discussion and treatment. Second, many patients hardly discuss their thoughts and rituals because the content is scatological or sexual, therefore, patients have to feel that the clinician will understand the anguish they experience and may be confident with the unacceptable content of their symptoms. Third, when treatments require a long period of testing, that can cause increased anxiety; the relationship with the clinician must be strong if the treatment is to be sustained. Fourth, since treatment is often not fully effective, many patients have a chronic course, so the relationship with the clinician can be long and must be able to sustain both parties.

After establishing the diagnosis, it is very important to sit down with the patient and their parents/spouses and review the causes, nature, and course of the disease. The clinician must explain the relevance of the comorbid characteristics to define the interventions and the prognosis of the disorder. This may need to be repeated several times during the course of treatment. It is useful for the patient and family to know the probable natural chronic course of OCD, the treatment objectives to reduce the interferences that cause the symptoms in the life of the patient, and the importance of ensuring an optimal development of the child. In addition, it is important to assist the family to learn how they can provide the best patient support and discover what support they need to sustain themselves for a long time. At the same time, clinicians have several reasons to be optimistic and encouraged about the fact that symptoms can be reduced.

The consensus is that behavioral treatments, particularly cognitive-behavioral therapy, are the first intervention strategy for children and adolescents whose symptoms are mild to moderate. Behavioral treatments have been systematically studied for children and adults. There are many reports of simple studies of cases without a control group. Behavioral techniques such as auto objection, extinction, operant conditioning, and modeling have been used with adolescents. The combination of implosion and prevention of response seems to produce favorable results with adolescents and adults who suffer from compulsions. This method uses direct and imaginary exposure to the feared object or events, followed by the frustration of any opportunity to engage in symptomatic reactions.

A patient with a fear of contamination by garbage would put their hands in a garbage can and would be restricted to wash for a period of hours. The improvement rates are 90%, achieving moderate to complete improvement and correlated with neuroanatomical changes. A variation of this technique that may be less applicable to children and adolescents, consists of a progressive exposure combined with prevention of response. March (1994) used cognitive-behavioral therapy combined with exposure and prevention of response in the treatment of 15 children, of which 9 (60%) obtained a reduction of at least 50% of the symptoms that was maintained for 18 months. De Haan (1998) found that exposure with prevention of response is as effective as treatment with clomipramine. Despite flaws in the designs, there is evidence of the usefulness of these techniques and the best results were obtained when trained and experienced people applied them. Clinicians who are trained and experienced in these techniques obtain the best results.

Pharmacological Potentiation

The failure of SSRI treatment is sometimes addressed by the addition of other drugs. There is evidence of some benefit when typical or atypical antipsychotics are used at low doses, in addition to SSRIs. It is estimated that there is a response in one-third of patients' refractory to SSRIs receiving antipsychotics, with a number needing to treat 4.6%, especially if there are tics such as comorbidity. No antipsychotic seems to be superior to the others, but haloperidol and risperidone are apparently very effective. Given that the profiles of adverse effects of SSRIs are more benign, at least 2 schemes of these drugs should be tried before attempting to potentiate them

Effects of Serotonin and Dopamine in Obsessive Compulsive Disorder with antipsychotics.

There is evidence that some polymorphisms in the gene that codes for an important neuronal transporter of glutamate are associated with OCD, and studies of spectroscopy and cerebrospinal fluid revealed alterations of the glutamatergic pathway in patients with this disease, so this neurotransmitter currently represents a therapeutic white interesting. Memantine is a low-affinity non-competitive blocker on the N-methyl-D-aspartate (NMDA) receptor that could be effective in treating adults and children with OCD, with a relatively benign profile of adverse effects. Glycine is a co-agonist of the NMDA receptor, and its use was superior to placebo in improving OCD symptoms, although it did not reach statistical significance. However, tolerance to this agent is very low. Sarcosine, a glycine reuptake inhibitor, was associated with a 20% reduction in OCD symptoms, while ketamine, a high potency NMDA blocker, has a rapid antidepressant effect from one day to 2 weeks, including in patients with major refractory depression to treatment and, possibly, in OCD (although in subjects with comorbidities and more severe disease, no benefit was observed). Other drugs that modulate glutamate and could be useful to treat OCD are riluzole, topiramate (with a greater effect on compulsions than obsessions, but many adverse effects), lamotrigine, and N-acetylcysteine (the latter two, especially, as SSRI enhancers). Other drugs that could have an effect to treat OCD are mirtazapine (seems to accelerate and improve the response to citalopram, compared with the latter and placebo), opioids (morphine was linked with improvement in the severity of OCD symptoms after 2 weeks, while tramadol would be useful to potentiate other drugs) and ondansetron (at low doses, it may relieve symptoms of OCD). Caffeine was associated with a significant improvement in patients' refractory to other OCD treatments, after 5 weeks of therapy.

Psychotherapy to Treat OCD

Behavioral therapy techniques have been especially effective in people with OCD who manifest the disease with compulsions, that is, with behaviors that are comparable to rituals. With this type of therapy, the patient is helped to face the idea, situation, or object that he fears, as well as to avoid the response, behavior, or ritual he adopts to defend himself from that fear. If the most important problem is obsessive thoughts; cognitive therapy may be the most appropriate option. This is because these thoughts are not the problem because all people can have them at some time, but it is the perception of the patient that those thoughts are a danger and are responsible for what may happen, and try to do something to feel safe and prevent this from happening.

Pharmacotherapy

Treatment with a single drug has been shown to be effective in almost 50% of patients. The first systematized investigations on medication were plagued with errors in diagnosis and measurements, which prevents the generalization and interpretation of data. Currently, a variety of substances with inhibitory properties of serotonin, seem to be useful in the treatment of OCD. Due to the fact that news about efficacy is present everywhere in advertisements and media, this can mistakenly lead patients to conclude that all OCD patients will be cured by medication. It is useful to explain to patients from the beginning that the most robust studies have shown that 40 to 50% of patients who have not received medication experience a 25-40% reduction in the severity of symptoms with treatment. This is important that consent is obtained before treatment and to help patients understand why they may continue to experience symptoms after a period of treatment. The choice of the most effective treatment will depend not only on the presence of OCD, but also on the other psychopathology present, such as psychotic or schizotypal characteristics, panic disorder, depression, or Tourette's. In order to determine if the patient responds to the medication, it must be administered in a dose and for a sufficient time. Most trials suggest that an adequate test would be when the patient receives the maximum allowable or tolerable dose for twelve weeks. Gradual reductions are strongly recommended when thinking about suspending medications with short half-lives such as fluvoxamine, paroxetine, and sertraline.

The drugs most fully studied in the treatment of OCD are the powerful SSRIs which also affect other neurotransmitter systems. Blinded, placebo-controlled trials have been performed in children with clomipramine, fluoxetine, fluvoxamine, and sertraline. Open trials with paroxetine and with citalopram have also been reported. With the advent of new federal government standards calling for safe and effective studies in children, clinicians can look forward to finding new agents outside of those already approved for use in children. There have been few comparative studies among these agents and this gives few clues to clinicians to make the first choice between them. One study attempted to predict the response to placebo or active agents by stratifying the cohort according to certain subgroups corresponding to some analyzed factors. Their results suggest that the subgroup with predominant symptoms of hoarding is less likely to respond to SSRIs than other OCD subtypes, observing that among the remaining subgroups there were no differences in their response.

In adolescent patients, clomipramine has been more studied. Initial studies report an average of 46% reduction of symptoms in 74% of patients. These results correlate with adult trials, where a reduction in symptoms of 30% is described. The improvement occurred in a wide variety of patients in both studies and was independent of the type of symptoms, the age of onset, or response to previous medication. Subsequently, it was found that the response correlates with the concentration of 5-HT and MAO activity; low concentration of 5-HT was associated with greater severity of symptoms and high concentration of 5-HT seems to predict clinical response to clomipramine. The specificity of the serotoninergic effects of clomipramine in the treatment of OCD symptoms was suggested by two studies. In a double-blinded, placebo-controlled study of desipramine vs clomipramine, desipramine was no more effective than placebo in reducing

OCD symptoms in adolescents. Then, in a double-blinded study of substitution, it suggested substantially higher relapse rates with desipramine, compared with clomipramine.

The side effects of clomipramine can be problematic. Anticholinergic effects including dizziness, xerostomia, blurred vision, postural hypotension, tachycardia, sedation, and constipation can occur and generate dissatisfaction. These effects can be avoided starting with very low doses and increasing very slowly until the reduction of symptoms is achieved. The maximum recommended dose is 5 mg/kg/day or 250 mg/day. It is recommended to perform electrocardiograms and liver function studies, with intervals of 3 months, during the adjustment of the dose and at least during the first year; subsequently, these controls must be done at least every 6 months. In adults, fewer side effects are reported with fluoxetine than with clomipramine. Double-blinded, placebo-controlled trials in children suggest that fluoxetine is effective in the control of OCD symptoms. The most commonly used initial doses are 5 mg/day and gradual increments up to a maximum of 60 mg/day. Of the side effects reported, the most frequent are agitation, insomnia, anorexia, dizziness, xerostomia, increased anxiety, and possibly akathisia. Concerns have been expressed about suicidal ideation and aggression.

Sertraline was reported as safe and useful in an open-label trial and therefore superior to placebo in a multi-center, double-blinded, placebo-controlled trial of 187 patients. Doses higher than 200 mg/day were administered in a flexible strategy. Using a definition of a 25% or greater reduction in symptoms, 42% of patients were considered responders. The response rate with placebo was 26%. Thirteen-percent of patients discontinued the medication due to side effects, among which listed as more common insomnia, nausea, agitation, and tremor. No effects were reported on vital signs or cardiac function. Fluvoxamine has a structure with only one ring. Collateral effects are reportedly less common and include nausea, lethargy, and insomnia. Doses start at 25 mg/day and gradually increase to a maximum of 5 mg/kg/day or 300 mg/day. In an open-label study, doses of 100-300 mg were used in 14 adolescents with OCD; nine of them (62%) had a reduction in the Y-BOCS scales of 8 points or more. Then a double-blinded study of Fluvoxamine was carried out using doses of up to 200 mg/day in 136 children and adolescents with OCD; the treatment produced an average of 25% (or greater) decrease in the CY-BOCS scale, after 10 weeks. Overall, 42% of patients were considered responders.

It can be easily seen that between 40% and 50% of people with OCD without associated diagnoses may not respond to adequate trials with SSRIs. The response to one SRI agent does not predict the response to another, and the side effects of one may not predict the collateral effects of another. For this reason, it is important to administer adequate doses for a sufficient period of time and at least two drugs of the same group before opting for potentiation strategies. When agents are combined with SSRIs, particular attention must be paid to the metabolism pathways of the agents used. Interactions based on inhibition of the cytochrome P-450 system can lead to side effects and toxicity. Before adding any prescription to an SSRI, there are excellent and reliable resources of websites that can be consulted.

Although the use of polypharmacy is generally avoided, when adequate trials with two drugs fail, potentiation strategies may be necessary. It was found that patients with Tourette, tics, or family history of tics that were refractory to treatment with a single SRI could benefit from the addition of a dopaminergic blocker such as haloperidol or pimozide. In addition, a few patients with refractory OCD to SRI, who have not had tics or a family history of tics, also improved with the addition of these same agents. This study was reproduced with risperidone and olanzapine considering its important results as well. Dopaminergic inhibition in the corticoestratothalomocortical circuit can be critical for the successful facilitation of 5-HT. There is little data on the addition of lithium or triiodothyronine. Buspirone may increase serotonergic activity in conjunction with SSRIs, but there was no evidence of the benefit of using an enhancement strategy with buspirone in OCD. Small-scale studies suggest that the addition of clomipramine to an SSRI may be justified. Maximum care should be taken in monitoring with electrocardiographic changes and collateral cardiovascular effects. Clonazepam has been useful to add in case of comorbid anxiety or panic, but sedation and memory problems may occur. Serious toxic effects result when combining fluoxetine with L-tryptophan, and therefore this mixture is discouraged.

Psychodynamic psychotherapy may be indicated when children have conflicts, associated with their obsessions or compulsions, which interfere with their optimal development. The use of psychodynamic psychotherapy for patients with OCD does not mean that a clinician has determined that OCD has a psychodynamic etiology. Psychodynamic treatment plays a role in the treatment of reactions or conflicts that accompany OCD. Example of this could include insecurities related to family dysfunction or divorce, deterioration of self-esteem, inappropriate expectations, perfectionist efforts, regulation of sexual and aggressive impulses, and the impact of a potentially chronic disease during the years of development. Patients can also adopt defenses that obstruct their recovery. By decreasing the impact of these impairments, psychotherapy can reduce the patient's tension and help in their treatment.

It is not necessary to hospitalize patients to assess their symptoms completely. In any case, patients and their families face a crisis when the spiral of symptoms becomes completely out of their control, the family's capacity to support the patient is almost exhausted, the symptoms are dangerous, or the course of an adequate treatment failure. Although these circumstances may pressure clinicians to initiate additional interventions quickly, it should be remembered that, usually, crises emerge from chronic stresses accumulated for a long time. Starting treatment without a sufficient understanding of these stresses can undermine subsequent therapy. During a crisis, the patient can benefit from hospitalization as an alternative to precipitate changes in outpatient treatment. Hospitalization can decrease the burden on parents/spouses to manage, contain uncontrollable symptoms, and reduce the patient's impossible requests for instant improvement. This reduces the risk of inappropriate interventions. The primary objectives of hospitalization are to quickly provide an objective assessment of the severity of the patient's deterioration outside the home; facilitate the simultaneous initiation of family, psychological and pharmacological treatments, and reduce symptoms reducing stress and anxiety.

Results and Follow Up

The outcome of an episode of OCD can range from complete and permanent recovery to inexorable deterioration. Points in this continuum include complete remission with discrete recurrent episodes, partial remission (mild to moderate chronic symptoms), and partial remission with occasional severe crises. Samples of self-referred patients for treatment cannot provide a generalizable conclusion about the results. Some researchers suggest that, in adults, a continuum of disease with fluctuating severity is more common (84%) and a course toward deterioration is the next most common

(15%). Others report 65% spontaneous remission rates of two continuous years. A cohort of 40 patients in treatment for two years was followed, discovering more than 80% improvement in all measures in the 37 available subjects. However, when hospitalized patients were sampled, the levels of great improvement decreased to 30%. Based on the reports of others, it was reported that the most common course of the disease was intermittent (remission of symptoms between episodes) (56%), although chronic disease (constant severity without remissions) was common (27%), just as it was an episodic course (single episode in the last five years or less) (17%).

There has been the challenge of obtaining solid longitudinal clinical data. This gap was reduced with a study on the natural history of 251 adults over 30 years. In this sample, 29% had their beginning of OCD before 20 years, 40% between 20 and 29 years and 23% after 30 years. These findings correspond to the other studies that reported 40% with onset before the age of 20 and the average age of beginning near 20 years. The ECA study also reflects this data, since the average age was between 20.9 and 25.4 years of age. In a prospective study of a clinical cohort of adolescents, Swedo (2012) evaluated 27 adolescents who participated in clomipramine clinical trials. Twenty-five seen 2-5 years subsequent to clinical trials, continued to experience anxiety or depression despite improvement in OCD. Bolton (2013) reviewed the results of 15 inpatient and outpatient adolescents 9-48 months after behavioral and family therapy. A good response to treatment was presented in 66%. Leonard (1993) reviewed the records of 54 adolescents at 3.5 (range 2-7) years after treatment. Although 94% had some symptoms, 57% did not fill criteria for OCD; 19% were worse than in the initial evaluation; 70% continued with medication. Poor response to medication, the presence of tics, and psychopathology of the parents predicted the poorer outcome (Leonard; 1992).

Recommendations

Benefits of Serotonin

The most important thing for one's health is to learn to conserve it! For this, you must begin by learning to establish a balance in all the biological processes of your body, which is why maintaining adequate levels of serotonin, can help a person.

Reconciling a restful sleep: serotonin for sleep

The correct blood levels of this chemical substance will allow you to achieve relaxation sensations that are conducive to rest, sleep, and rest of the mind and body; therefore, start a new day with a lot of positive energy.

Help in digestion

Nowadays, thanks to advances in science, it is proven that the highest amount of serotonin can be located in the digestive system; the balance in the levels of this substance will help to make a correct digestion of food, avoiding an irritable colon and intestinal pains.

Reduces the risk of obesity

Serotonin gives the body a sensation of relaxation when eating, so you will feel satiety consuming small amounts of food, in the same way, the correct levels of serotonin fights anxiety, thus then avoiding the consumption of foods that are conducive to weight gain.

Prevents premature skin aging

Because serotonin produces a large amount of antioxidants, it makes it easier for the skin to eliminate dead cells, thus achieving rejuvenation.

Relieves stress and anxiety

Serotonin, in nocturnal hours, favors the production of sleep and allows total relaxation. During those moments, the brain allows you to approach those situations from a second plane and decide the reactions that most favor you.

Serotonin low in blood

It is important that if your doctor indicates whether one

should perform an exam to determine your serum level, that is, to know your serotonin levels in the blood, identifying the symptoms is of vital importance to determine whether or not you need this test. An individual should always remember that the main goal is to maintain an optimal state of health, paying attention to the signals that their body sends to them. If a person regularly has insomnia, anxiety, or gets depressed easily, the cause is probably low levels of serotonin, but the doctor is the one to guide the person as it could also be a symptom of many other conditions.

Physical and emotional symptoms

The identification of what serotonin produces in one's mind and body is the first task to regulate their levels and have a better quality of life. There are some physical symptoms showing that this substance is produced in one's body:

1. Regularize positive and negative states of mind: Once regularized in your body the levels of this substance are the only ones that decide how to present yourself to

other people, it is your task to show that you can deal with situations that generate stress without losing patience. Always a positive vision of what surrounds you.

2. <u>Controls the level of body temperature</u>: Serotonin is responsible for the thermal regulation of our body, i.e. when we present fevers due to any disease, serotonin then begins a fight with that factor that generates the elevation of the temperature of your body.

3. <u>Influences sexual desire</u>: This chemical is designed to fulfill the function of providing your body with sensations that generate pleasure and relaxation, which is why the desire and subsequent sexual activity favor the serotonin standards.

Causes and consequences

To identify which are the factors that influence in keeping serotonin low is very important, which is why a person should know the following:

1. Feeding of sugars and processed flours favors the production of anaerobic bacteria that alter the bacterial flora in the intestines. This affects bacteria that without helping the process of food digestion, constipation occurs and the absorption of tryptophan is not achieved, which is an amino acid that is given to us through the consumption of meat, bananas, and milk. This causes that the alteration of the intestinal flora does not allow the synthesis of serotonin, thus preventing it from reaching the nervous system correctly.

2. Stress, in many cases, causes people to live the day-to-day exhausted, irritable, and with mood swings; this state produces a hormone called cortisol, which recent studies have shown that produces a toxic action on the brain. Then we can infer that the presence of cortisol gives the brain unfavorable conditions and serotonin in particular decreases considerably in the presence of cortisol.

Future Investigations

There are a series of factors or characteristics in each patient that can favor a better or worse response to treatment. However, the failure of the same usually occurs in patients who do not meet the indications of the therapist; in those who have a depression or severe anxiety associated, as well as when they consume alcohol or drugs, have a low IQ or present alterations of personality or difficulties for relationships with other people. Researchers have remained optimistic about clinical care. The interest in OCD has produced well-informed clinicians with greater skills for diagnosis and treatment. Self-help organizations open the possibility of public information and alleviate the loneliness of many people with OCD. As organizations and clinicians inform the public, people who feared treatment or have had disappointments with previous efforts, can receive treatment, benefit from new knowledge and receive some relief. The use of specific behavioral techniques, treatments of dynamically informed families, psychotherapy, and medication, can now offer improvement for the majority of seriously ill patients.

    Pharmacological treatments, even with potentiation, are not yet effective enough for up to 40% of patients suffering from OCD, especially for those with the prominence of hoarding symptoms. Apparently, many people with OCD continue to suffer in secret. Epidemiological studies remind us that many patients with OCD have not searched or been treated. There are too few clinicians specifically trained in cognitive-behavioral treatment techniques and there is a tendency to neglect this intervention. Continuous and vigorous efforts are still needed for the public to be informed and to attend a clinical examination to diagnose OCD. As we learn more about neural circuits and the chemical functioning of the brain, there will be a realistic basis for hope that new and better treatments will become available for the future years. In addition, preventive measures can help reduce the risk of developing OCD and the severity of its symptoms once the genetic factors are known.

9 REFERENCES

Alevizos, B., Lykouras, L., Zervas, I. M., & Christodoulou, G. N. (2002). Risperidone-induced obsessive compulsive symptoms: A series of six cases. Journal of Clinical Psychopharmacology, 22(5), 461-467. Retrieved from SCOPUS database.

American Psychiatric Association. (2000). Diagnostic and statistical manual of mental disorders. 4th edition, text revision (DSM-IV-TR). Washington, DC: American Psychiatric Association,

American Psychiatric Association. (July 2007). [Guideline] American psychiatric association workgroup on obsessive compulsive disorder. practice guideline for the treatment of patients with obsessive compulsive disorder. Am J Psychiatry, 164(suppl), 1-56.

Aouizerate, B., Cuny, E., Martin-Guehl, C., Guehl, D., Amieva, H., Benazzouz, A., et al. (2004). Deep brain stimulation of the ventral caudate nucleus in the treatment of obsessive compulsive disorder and major depression:

Case report. Journal of Neurosurgery, 101(4), 682-686. doi:10.3171/jns.2004.101.4.0682

Aouizerate, B., Guehl, D., Cuny, E., Rougier, A., Bioulac, B., Tignol, J., et al. (2004). Pathophysiology of obsessive compulsive disorder: A necessary link between phenomenology, neuropsychology, imagery and physiology. Progress in Neurobiology, 72(3), 195-221. Retrieved from SCOPUS database.

Arntz, A., Voncken, M., & Goosen, A. C. A. (2007). Responsibility and obsessive- compulsive disorder: An experimental test. Behaviour Research and Therapy, 45(3), 425-435. Retrieved from SCOPUS database.

Bergqvist, P. B. F., Dong, J., & Blier, P. (1999). Effect of atypical antipsychotic drugs on 5-HT2 receptors in the rat orbito-frontal cortex: An in vivo electrophysiological study. Psychopharmacology, 143(1), 89-96. Retrieved from SCOPUS database.

Berridge, K. C., Aldridge, J. W., Houchard, K. R., & Zhuang, X. (2005). Sequential super- stereotypy of an instinctive fixed action pattern in hyper-dopaminergic mutant mice: A model of obsessive compulsive disorder and tourette's. BMC Biol, 3, 4.

Besson, M., Belin, D., McNamara, R., Theobald, D. E. H., Castel, A., Beckett, V. L., et al. (2010). Dissociable control of impulsivity in rats by dopamine D2/3 receptors in the core and shell subregions of the nucleus accumbens. Neuropsychopharmacology, 35(2), 560-569. Retrieved from SCOPUS database.

Björgvinsson, T., Hart, J., & Heffelfinger, S. (2007). Obsessive compulsive disorder: Update on assessment and treatment. Journal of Psychiatric Practice, 13(6), 362-372. doi:10.1097/01.pra.0000300122.76322.ad

Blier, P., Habib, R., & Flament, M. F. (2006). Pharmacotherapies in the management of obsessive compulsive disorder. Canadian Journal of Psychiatry, 51(7), 417-430. Retrieved from SCOPUS database.

Boulougouris, V., Chamberlain, S. R., & Robbins, T. W. (2009). Cross-species models of OCD spectrum disorders. Psychiatry Research, 170(1), 15-21. doi:10.1016/j.psychres.2008.07.016

Brown, S. A., Crowell-Davis, S., Malcolm, T., & Edwards, P. (1987). Naloxone-responsive compulsive tail chasing in a dog. J Am Vet Med Assoc, 190(7), 884-6.

Campbell, K. M., De Lecea, L., Severynse, D. M., Caron, M. G., McGrath, M. J., Sparber, S. B., et al. (1999). OCD-like behaviors caused by a neuropotentiating transgene targeted to cortical and limbic D1+ neurons. Journal of Neuroscience, 19(12), 5044- 5053. Retrieved from SCOPUS database.

Choi, Y. -. (2009). Efficacy of treatments for patients with obsessive compulsive disorder: A systematic review. Journal of the American Academy of Nurse Practitioners, 21(4), 207-213. doi:10.1111/j.1745-7599.2009.00408.x

Chou-Green, J. M., Holscher, T. D., Dallman, M. F., & Akana, S. F. (2003). Compulsive behavior in the 5-HT2C receptor knockout mouse. Physiol Behav, 78(4-5), 641-9.

Davidson, J., & Bjorgvinsson, T. (2003). Current and potential pharmacological treatments for obsessive compulsive disorder. Expert Opinion on Investigational Drugs, 12(6), 993-1001. Retrieved from SCOPUS database.

Dell'Osso, B., Buoli, M., Baldwin, D. S., & Altamura, A. C. (2010). Serotonin norepinephrine reuptake inhibitors (SNRIs) in anxiety disorders: A comprehensive review of their clinical efficacy. Human Psychopharmacology, 25(1), 17-29. Retrieved from SCOPUS database.

Dell'Osso, B., Nestadt, G., Allen, A., & Hollander, E. (2006). Serotonin-norepinephrine reuptake inhibitors in the treatment of obsessive compulsive disorder: A critical review. Journal of Clinical Psychiatry, 67(4), 600-610. Retrieved from SCOPUS database.

den Heuvel, O. A. v., der Werf, Y. D. v., Verhoef, K. M. W., de Wit, S., Berendse, H. W., Wolters, E. C., et al. (2010).

Frontal-striatal abnormalities underlying behaviours in the compulsive-impulsive spectrum. Journal of the Neurological Sciences, 289(1-2), 55-59. Retrieved from SCOPUS database.

Denys, D., Klompmakers, A. A., & Westenberg, H. G. M. (2004). Synergistic dopamine increase in the rat prefrontal cortex with the combination of quetiapine and fluvoxamine. Psychopharmacology, 176(2), 195-203. doi:10.1007/s00213-004- 1880-0

Denys, D., Van Der Wee, N., Janssen, J., De Geus, F., & Westenberg, H. G. M. (2004). Low level of dopaminergic D2 receptor binding in obsessive compulsive disorder. Biological Psychiatry, 55(10), 1041-1045. Retrieved from SCOPUS database.

Denys, D., Zohar, J., & Westenberg, H. G. M. (2004). The role of dopamine in obsessive- compulsive disorder: Preclinical and clinical evidence. Journal of Clinical Psychiatry, 65(SUPPL. 14), 11-17. Retrieved from SCOPUS database.

Dougherty, D. D., Rauch, S. L., & Jenike, M. A. (2004). Pharmacotherapy for obsessive- compulsive disorder. Journal of Clinical Psychology, 60(11), 1195-1202. Retrieved from SCOPUS database.

Eagle, D. M., Lehmann, O., Theobald, D. E. H., Pena, Y., Zakaria, R., Ghosh, R., et al. (2009). Serotonin depletion impairs waiting but not stop-signal reaction time in rats: Implications for theories of the role of 5-HT in behavioral inhibition. Neuropsychopharmacology, 34(5), 1311-1321. doi:10.1038/npp.2008.202

El Mansari, M., & Blier, P. (2006). Mechanisms of action of current and potential pharmacotherapies of obsessive compulsive disorder. Progress in Neuro-Psychopharmacology and Biological Psychiatry, 30(3), 362-373. Retrieved from SCOPUS database.

El Mansari, M., Bouchard, C., & Blier, P. (1995). Alteration of serotonin release in the guinea pig orbito-frontal cortex by selective serotonin reuptake inhibitors. relevance to treatment of obsessive compulsive disorder.

Neuropsychopharmacology, 13(2), 117-127. Retrieved from SCOPUS database.

Fineberg, N. A., Potenza, M. N., Chamberlain, S. R., Berlin, H. A., Menzies, L., Bechara, A., et al. (2010). Probing compulsive and impulsive behaviors, from animal models to endophenotypes: A narrative review. Neuropsychopharmacology, 35(3), 591-604. Retrieved from SCOPUS database.

Goddard, A. W., Shekhar, A., Whiteman, A. F., & McDougle, C. J. (2008). Serotoninergic mechanisms in the treatment of obsessive compulsive disorder. Drug Discovery Today, 13(7-8), 325-332. Retrieved from SCOPUS database.

Goodman, W. K., Barr, L. C., McDougle, C. J., & Price, L. H. (1993). Beyond the serotonin hypothesis of OCD. European Neuropsychopharmacology, 3(3), 229. Retrieved from SCOPUS database.

Goodman, W. K., Price, L. H., Rasmussen, S. A., Mazure, C., Delgado, P., Heninger, G. R., et al. (1989). The yale-brown obsessive compulsive scale. II. validity.

Archives of General Psychiatry, 46(11), 1012-1016. Retrieved from SCOPUS database.

Goodman, W. K., Price, L. H., Rasmussen, S. A., Mazure, C., Fleischmann, R. L., Hill, C. L., et al. (1989). The yale-brown obsessive compulsive scale. I. development, use and reliability. Archives of General Psychiatry, 46(11), 1006-1011. Retrieved from SCOPUS database.

Greer, J. M., & Capecchi, M. R. (2002). Hoxb8 is required for normal grooming behavior in mice. Neuron, 33(1), 23-34.

Grindlinger, H. M., & Ramsay, E. (1991). Compulsive feather picking in birds. Arch Gen Psychiatry, 48(9), 857.

Hollander, E. (2005). Obsessive compulsive disorder and spectrum across the life span. International Journal of Psychiatry in Clinical Practice, 9(2), 79-86. Retrieved from SCOPUS database.

Jackson, C. W., Morton, W. A., & Lydiard, R. B. (1994). Pharmacologic management of obsessive compulsive disorder. Southern Medical Journal, 87(3), 310-321. Retrieved from SCOPUS database.

Joel, D., & Avisar, A. (2001). Excessive lever pressing following post-training signal attenuation in rats: A possible animal model of obsessive compulsive disorder? Behavioural Brain Research, 123(1), 77-87. Retrieved from SCOPUS database.

Joel, D., & Doljansky, J. (2003). Selective alleviation of compulsive lever-pressing in rats by D1, but not D2, blockade: Possible implications for the involvement of D1 receptors in obsessive compulsive disorder. Neuropsychopharmacology : Official Publication of the American College of Neuropsychopharmacology, 28(1), 77-85. Retrieved from SCOPUS database.

Joel, D., Doljansky, J., Roz, N., & Rehavi, M. (2005). Role of the orbital cortex and of the serotonergic system in a rat model of obsessive compulsive disorder. Neuroscience,

130(1), 25-36. Retrieved from SCOPUS database.

Joel, D., Doljansky, J., & Schiller, D. (2005). 'Compulsive' lever pressing in rats is enhanced following lesions to the orbital cortex, but not to the basolateral nucleus of the amygdala or to the dorsal medial prefrontal cortex. European Journal of Neuroscience, 21(8), 2252-2262. Retrieved from SCOPUS database.

Katz, R. J. (1991). Neurobiology of obsessive compulsive disorder - A serotonergic basis of freudian repression. Neuroscience and Biobehavioral Reviews, 15(3), 375-381. Retrieved from SCOPUS database.

Kopell, B. H., Greenberg, B., & Rezai, A. R. (2004). Deep brain stimulation for psychiatric disorders. Journal of Clinical Neurophysiology, 21(1), 51-67. doi:10.1097/00004691 200401000-00007

Leckman, J. F., Goodman, W. K., North, W. G., Chappell, P. B., Price, L. H., Pauls, D. L., et al. (1994). Elevated cerebrospinal fluid levels of oxytocin in obsessive compulsive disorder: Comparison with tourette's syndrome and healthy controls. Archives of General Psychiatry, 51(10), 782-792. Retrieved from SCOPUS database.

Lochner, C., & Stein, D. J. (2006). Does work on obsessive compulsive spectrum disorders contribute to understanding the heterogeneity of obsessive compulsive disorder? Progress in Neuro-Psychopharmacology and Biological Psychiatry, 30(3), 353-361. Retrieved from SCOPUS database.

Luescher, U. A., McKeown, D. B., & Dean, H. (1998). A cross-sectional study on compulsive behaviour (stable vices) in horses. Equine Vet J Suppl, (27), 14-8.

Markarian, Y., Larson, M. J., Aldea, M. A., Baldwin, S. A., Good, D., Berkeljon, A., et al. (2010). Multiple pathways to functional impairment in obsessive compulsive disorder. Clinical Psychology Review, 30(1), 78-88. Retrieved from SCOPUS database.

Math, S. B., & Janardhan Reddy, Y. C. (2007). Issues in the pharmacological treatment of obsessive compulsive disorder. International Journal of Clinical Practice, 61(7), 1188-1197. doi:10.1111/j.1742-1241.2007.01356.x

Matsunaga, H., Nagata, T., Hayashida, K., Ohya, K., Kiriike, N., & Stein, D. J. (2009). A long-term trial of the effectiveness and safety of atypical antipsychotic agents in augmenting SSRI-refractory obsessive compulsive disorder. Journal of Clinical Psychiatry, 70(6), 863-868. Retrieved from SCOPUS database.

Meck, W. H. (2006). Neuroanatomical localization of an internal clock: A functional link between mesolimbic, nigrostriatal, and mesocortical dopaminergic systems. Brain Research, 1109(1), 93-107. Retrieved from SCOPUS database.

Nuttin, B. J., Gabriëls, L. A., Cosyns, P. R., Meyerson, B. A., Andréewitch, S., Sunaert, S. G., et al. (2008). Long-term electrical capsular stimulation in patients with obsessive compulsive disorder. Neurosurgery, 62(6 SUPPL.) doi:10.1227/01.NEU.0000064565.49299.9A

Olver, J. S., O'Keefe, G., Jones, G. R., Burrows, G. D., Tochon-Danguy, H. J., Ackermann, U., et al. (2009). Dopamine D1 receptor binding in the striatum of patients with obsessive compulsive disorder. Journal of Affective Disorders, 114(1- 3), 321-326. Retrieved from SCOPUS database.

Olver, J. S., O'Keefe, G., Jones, G. R., Burrows, G. D., Tochon-Danguy, H. J., Ackermann, U., et al. (2010). Dopamine D1 receptor binding in the anterior cingulate cortex of patients with obsessive compulsive disorder. Psychiatry Research - Neuroimaging, 183(1), 85-88. Retrieved from SCOPUS database.

Phillipson, S. (2010). Guilt beyond a reasonable doubt. Retrieved 25th July, 2010, from http://www.ocdonline.com/articlephillipson2.php

Pogarell, O., Poepperl, G., Mulert, C., Hamann, C., Sadowsky, N., Riedel, M., et al. (2005). SERT and DAT availabilities under citalopram treatment in obsessive- compulsive disorder (OCD). European Neuropsychopharmacology,

15(5), 521-524. Retrieved from SCOPUS database.

Pum, M., Carey, R. J., Huston, J. P., & Müller, C. P. (2007). Dissociating effects of cocaine and d-amphetamine on dopamine and serotonin in the perirhinal, entorhinal, and prefrontal cortex of freely moving rats. Psychopharmacology, 193(3), 375-390. Retrieved from SCOPUS database.

Puumala, T., & Sirviö, J. (1998). Changes in activities of dopamine and serotonin systems in the frontal cortex underlie poor choice accuracy and impulsivity of rats in an attention task. Neuroscience, 83(2), 489-499. Retrieved from SCOPUS database.

Ramesh Kumar, T. C., & Khanna, S. (2000). Lamotrigine augmentation of serotonin re- uptake inhibitors in obsessive compulsive disorder. Australian and New Zealand Journal of Psychiatry, 34(3), 527-528. Retrieved from SCOPUS database.

Rauch, S. L., Dougherty, D. D., Malone, D., Rezai, A., Friehs, G., Fischman, A. J., et al. (2006). A functional neuroimaging investigation of deep brain stimulation in patients with obsessive compulsive disorder. Journal of Neurosurgery, 104(4), 558-565.

doi:10.3171/jns.2006.104.4.558

Ravindran, A. V., Da Silva, T. L., Ravindran, L. N., Richter, M. A., & Rector, N. A. (2009). Obsessive compulsive spectrum disorders: A review of the evidence-based treatments. Canadian Journal of Psychiatry, 54(5), 331-343. Retrieved from SCOPUS database.

Robbins, T. W. (2002). The 5-choice serial reaction time task: Behavioural pharmacology and functional neurochemistry. Psychopharmacology, 163(3-4), 362-380. Retrieved from SCOPUS database.

Salamone, J. D., Correa, M., Mingote, S. M., & Weber, S. M. (2005). Beyond the reward hypothesis: Alternative functions of nucleus accumbens dopamine. Current Opinion in Pharmacology, 5(1), 34-41. Retrieved from SCOPUS database.

Schilman, E. A., Klavir, O., Winter, C., Sohr, R., & Joel, D. (2010). The role of the striatum in compulsive behavior in intact and orbitofrontal-cortex-lesioned rats: Possible involvement of the serotonergic system. Neuropsychopharmacology, 35(4), 1026-1039. Retrieved from SCOPUS database.

, S. (2008). Responsibility and impulsivity and their interaction in relation to obsessive compulsive symptoms. Journal of Behavior Therapy and Experimental Psychiatry, 39(3), 228-233. Retrieved from SCOPUS database.

Swanepoel, N., Lee, E., & Stein, D. J. (1998). Psychogenic alopecia in a cat: Response to clomipramine. J S Afr Vet Assoc, 69(1), 22.

Szechtman, H., Eckert, M. J., Tse, W. S., Boersma, J. T., Bonura, C. A., McClelland, J. Z., et al. (2001). Compulsive checking behavior of quinpirole-sensitized rats as an animal model of obsessive compulsive disorder(OCD): Form and control. BMC Neuroscience [Electronic

Resource], 2(1), 4. Retrieved from SCOPUS database.

Szechtman, H., Sulis, W., & Eilam, D. (1998). Quinpirole induces compulsive checking behavior in rats: A potential animal model of obsessive compulsive disorder (OCD). Behavioral Neuroscience, 112(6), 1475-1485. doi:10.1037/0735-7044.112.6.1475

Thoren, P., Asberg, M., & Bertilsson, L. (1980). Clomipramine treatment of obsessive- compulsive disorder. II. biochemical aspects. Archives of General Psychiatry, 37(11), 1289-1294. Retrieved from SCOPUS database.

Tizabi, Y., Louis, V. A., Taylor, C. T., Waxman, D., Culver, K. E., & Szechtman, H. (2002). Effect of nicotine on quinpirole-induced checking behavior in rats: Implications for obsessive compulsive disorder. Biological Psychiatry, 51(2), 164- 171. doi:10.1016/S0006-3223(01)01207-0

van Kuyck, K., Brak, K., Das, J., Rizopoulos, D., & Nuttin, B. (2008). Comparative study of the effects of electrical stimulation in the nucleus accumbens, the mediodorsal thalamic nucleus and the bed nucleus of the stria terminalis in rats with schedule- induced polydipsia. Brain Res, 1201, 93-9.

Weber, M., Talmon, S., Schulze, I., Boeddinghaus, C., Gross, G., Schoemaker, H., et al. (2009). Running wheel activity is sensitive to acute treatment with selective inhibitors for either serotonin or norepinephrine reuptake. Psychopharmacology, 203(4), 753-762. doi:10.1007/s00213-008-1420-4

Winstanley, C. A., Theobald, D. E. H., Dalley, J. W., & Robbins, T. W. (2005). Interactions between serotonin and dopamine in the control of impulsive choice in rats: Therapeutic implications for impulse control disorders. Neuropsychopharmacology, 30(4), 669-682. Retrieved from SCOPUS database.

Woods, A., Smith, C., Szewczak, M., Dunn, R. W., Cornfeldt, M., & Corbett, R. (1993). Selective serotonin re-uptake inhibitors decrease schedule-induced polydipsia in rats: A potential model for obsessive compulsive disorder.

Psychopharmacology, 112(2-3), 195-198. Retrieved from SCOPUS database.

Yin, H. H., & Knowlton, B. J. (2006). The role of the basal ganglia in habit formation. Nature Reviews Neuroscience, 7(6), 464-476. Retrieved from SCOPUS database.

Zeeb, F. D., Floresco, S. B., & Winstanley, C. A. (2010). Contributions of the orbitofrontal cortex to impulsive choice: Interactions with basal levels of impulsivity, dopamine signalling, and reward-related cues. Psychopharmacology, , 1-12. Retrieved from SCOPUS database.

Zhang, W., Perry, K. W., Wong, D. T., Potts, B. D., Bao, J., Tollefson, G. D., et al. (2000). Synergistic effects of olanzapine and other antipsychotic agents in combination with fluoxetine on norepinephrine and dopamine release in rat prefrontal cortex. Neuropsychopharmacology, 23(3), 250-262. doi:10.1016/S0893- 133X(00)00119-6

Zohar, J., Chopra, M., Sasson, Y., Amiaz, R., & Amital, D. (2000). Obsessive compulsive disorder: Serotonin and beyond. The World Journal of Biological Psychiatry : The Official Journal of the World Federation of Societies of Biological Psychiatry, 1(2), 92- 100. Retrieved from SCOPUS database.

ABOUT THE AUTHOR

A daughter, sister, niece, wife, mother, friend, and scientist. A graduate from the University of Florida (Go Gators!) in Animal Science, Business and Zoology; followed by a graduate degree also from the University of Florida in Clinical Research (Human Subjects); and subsequently, a PhD in Biological Sciences.